CONTENTS

CONTENTS

Abbreviations 4

Acknowledgements 5

Executive summary. 7

Key points 11

I. Introduction: Malaria outside of Africa is a disease of poverty that poses unique challenges for control 17

II. Global overview of malaria epidemiology 21
    Box 2.1: Comparison of P. falciparum *and* P. vivax *malaria* 23
    Box 2.2: Diagnosing P. falciparum *and* P. vivax 24
    Box 2.3: Comparison of some important vectors outside of Africa 29

III. South and South-East Asia 33
    Box 3.1: Malaria in the plains and forests of Orissa, India 39
    Box 3.2: Aiming to eliminate malaria in Bhutan 42
    Box 3.3: Resistance to antimalarial medicines and the insecticides used to control mosquitoes . 46
    Box 3.4: Asian Collaborative Training Network for Malaria. 47

IV. Oceania 49
    Box 4.1: Endemic and epidemic malaria in Papua New Guinea 53
    Box 4.2: Asia Pacific Malaria Elimination Network 55

V. The Americas 57
    Box 5.1: Malaria control in Suriname 61
    Box 5.2: The Amazon Malaria Initiative 65

VI. The Arabian Peninsula, the Caucasus and North-West Asia. 69
    Box 6.1. Delivering ITNs in Afghanistan 75

VII. Reducing malaria brings success and new challenges 79
    Box 7.1: Outbreaks and epidemics 82

VIII. Malaria programme response to new challenges 83

IX. The way forward 87

X. Conclusion 93

References 95

ABBREVIATIONS

ACD	Active case detection
ACT	Artemisinin-based combination therapy
ACTMalaria	Asian Collaborative Training Network for Malaria
AMI	Amazon Malaria Initiative
ANC	Antenatal care
APMEN	Asia Pacific Malaria Elimination Network
ASHA	Accredited social health activist
GF	The Global Fund to Fight AIDS, Tuberculosis and Malaria
G6PD	Glucose-6-phosphate dehydrogenase
IRS	Indoor residual spraying
ITN	Insecticide-treated mosquito net
LLIN	Long-lasting insecticidal net
MSD	Malaria service deliverers
NGO	Nongovernmental organization
NMLCP	National Malaria and Leishmaniasis Control Programme
NRHM	National Rural Health Mission
PATH	Program for Appropriate Technology in Health
PCR	Polymerase chain reaction
RBM	Roll Back Malaria
RDT	Rapid diagnostic test
RITM	Research Institute for Tropical Medicine
VDCP	Vector-borne Disease Control Programme
WHO	World Health Organization
WPRO	WHO Western Pacific Region

ROLL BACK MALARIA PARTNERSHIP

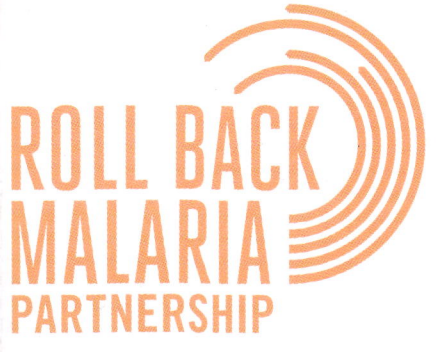

PROGRESS & IMPACT SERIES

Number 9 · November 2012

Defeating malaria in Asia, the Pacific, Americas, Middle East and Europe

World Health Organization

PATH
A catalyst for global health

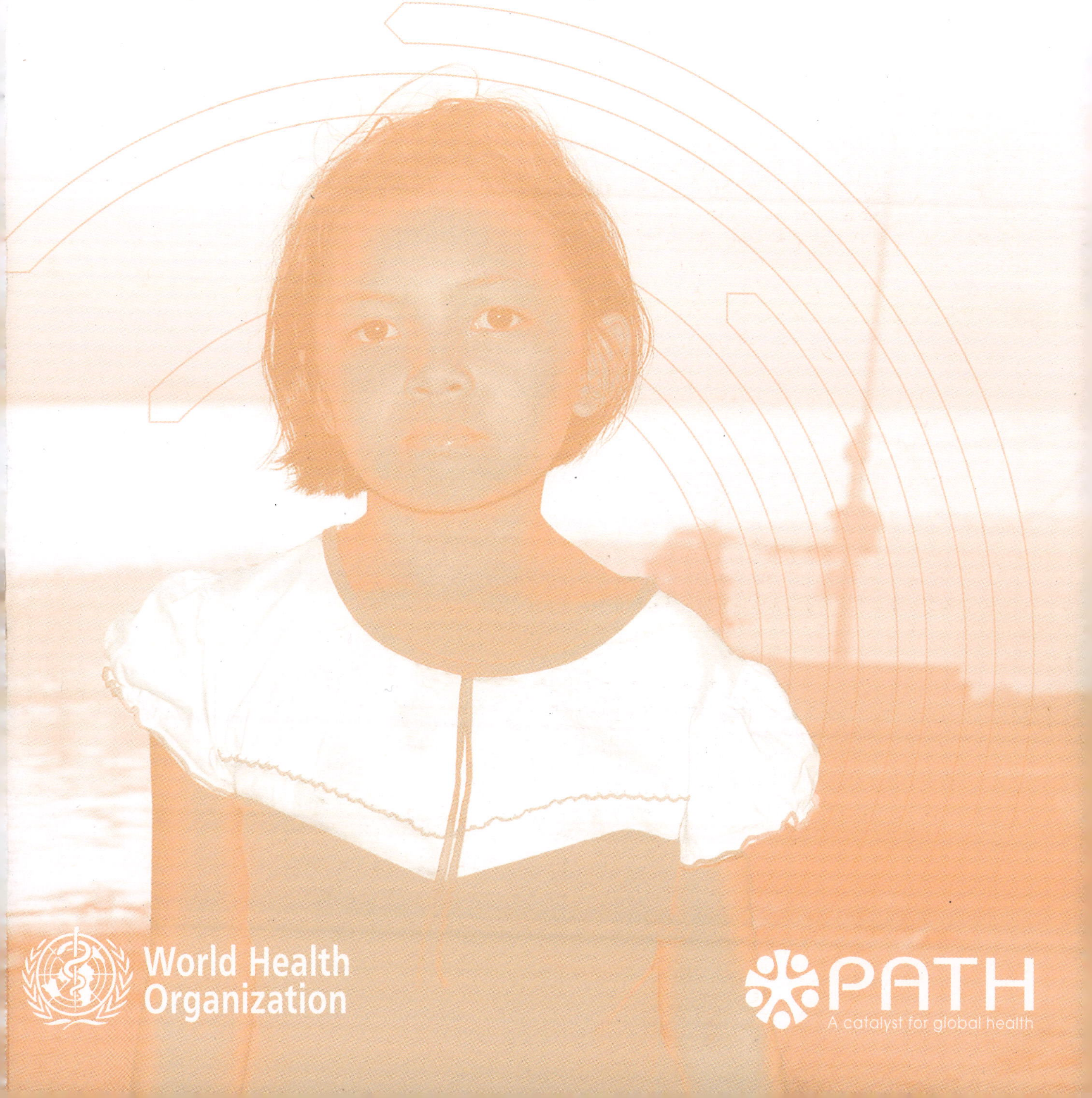

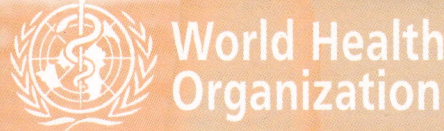

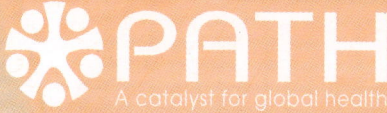

WHO Library Cataloguing-in-Publication Data

Defeating malaria in Asia, the Pacific, Americas, Middle East and Europe.
(Progress & Impact Series, n. 9)

2 v.

Contents: v. 1: Briefing for policy-makers -- v. 2: Technical report

1.Malaria - prevention and control. 2.Malaria - epidemiology. 3.International cooperation. 4.Asia. 5.Pacific Islands. 6.Americas. 7.Middle East. 8.Europe. I.Global Partnership to Roll Back Malaria. II.Series.

ISBN 978 92 4 150443 0   (NLM classification: WC 765)

© 2012 World Health Organization on behalf of the Roll Back Malaria Partnership Secretariat

All rights reserved. Requests for permission to reproduce or translate WHO publications – whether for sale or for noncommercial distribution – should be directed to the Roll Back Malaria (RBM) Partnership Secretariat at the address listed at the bottom of this page. Some photographs are subject to licensing fees and may not be reproduced freely; all photo enquiries should also be directed to the Secretariat.

The designations employed and the presentation of the material in this publication do not imply the expression of any opinion whatsoever on the part of the World Health Organization (WHO), the RBM Partnership Secretariat or any of its individual partners concerning the legal status of any country, territory, city or area or of its authorities, or concerning the delimitation of its frontiers or boundaries. Dotted lines on maps, where present, represent approximate border lines for which there may not yet be full agreement.

The data provided in this report were assembled from 2000 through 2011. Due to the constant updating of intervention coverage and the information supplied by countries and agencies, some numbers in this report may have since changed for this time interval; not all numbers are adjusted to a single date. However, such changes are generally minor and do not, at the time of publication, affect the overall picture of malaria intervention coverage and observed or estimated impact.

The mention or appearance in photographs of certain manufacturers and/or their products does not imply that they are endorsed or recommended by WHO, the RBM Partnership Secretariat or any of its individual partners in preference to others of a similar nature that are not mentioned.

Although every effort has been made to ensure accuracy, the information in this publication is being distributed without warranty of any kind, either expressed or implied. In no event shall WHO, the Secretariat or any of its individual partners be liable for any damages incurred arising from its use.

The named authors alone are responsible for the views expressed in this publication.

Maps | Ryan Williams, WHO Global Malaria Programme | Florence Rusciano, WHO Public Health Information and Geographic Information Systems.

Photo credits | Front cover: © Zoltan Balogh/WHO | pp. 6, 9, 10, 16, 20, 28, 32, 38, 44, 56, 67, 80, 92, 94: © John Rae/The Global Fund | p. 48: © Stefan Hoyer/WHO | p. 63: © Ministry of Health Malaria Program in Suriname | pp. 68, 91: © Christopher Black/WHO | pp. 78, 85, 86: © Stephenie Hollyman/WHO

Enquiries | Roll Back Malaria Partnership Secretariat | Hosted by the World Health Organization | Avenue Appia 20 | 1211 Geneva 27 | Switzerland | Tel.: +41 22 791 5869 | Fax: +41 22 791 1587 | E-mail: inforbm@who.int

Designed by ENLASO | Printed in France

ACKNOWLEDGEMENTS

This report was prepared under the auspices of the Roll Back Malaria (RBM) Partnership to help assess progress towards targets set out in the Global Malaria Action Plan and the Millennium Development Goals.

This report was co-authored by Richard Cibulskis of the World Health Organization (WHO) Global Malaria Programme and Roly Gosling, formerly of WHO and now with the Global Health Group [GHG], University of California, San Francisco [UCSF]. Maps of parasite prevalence were produced by the Malaria Atlas Project at the University of Oxford, while maps of disease distribution were produced by Ryan Williams of the WHO Global Malaria Programme.

The authors acknowledge with thanks the contributions of the many people who have participated in the collection and analysis of country information that is included in this report: Eric Mouzin (Roll Back Malaria [RBM] Partnership Secretariat); Arna Chancelor and Maxine Whitaker (Asia Pacific Malaria Elimination Network [APMEN]); Dawran Faizan (HealthNet); Jamie Chang (United States Agency for International Development [USAID]); Nancy Fullman, Allison Phillips, and Cara Smith Gueye (GHG, UCSF); Sami Hahzat (National Malaria Control Programme [NMCP], Afghanistan); Hélène Hiwat-Van Laar (Ministry of Health [MoH], Suriname); Cecil Hugo, Rogelio Mendoza, and Jufel Sebial (ACT Malaria); Leopoldo Villegas (ICF International); and Ghasem Zamani (WHO).

The following individuals reviewed the report and provided important assistance and feedback: Maru Aregawi, Amy Barrett, Andrea Bosman, Jo Lines, Shiva Murugasampillay, Robert Newman, Aafje Rietveld, Pascal Ringwald, Zsofia Szilagyi, and Ryan Williams (WHO Global Malaria Programme), Joelle Brown (University of California, Los Angeles), Fawzia Rasheed (Global Fund to Fight AIDS, Tuberculosis and Malaria), Chris Cotter (GHG, UCSF), Richard Steketee (the Malaria Control and Evaluation Partnership in Africa [MACEPA], a programme at PATH), Jimee Hwang (US Centers for Disease Control and Prevention, USA), and Simon Hay, Peter Gething, and Carlos Guerra (Malaria Atlas Project, Oxford University).

We thank the following people for their managerial support and their work on the production of the report: Cristina Herdman (MACEPA) was the production manager and lead editor; Manny Lewis (MACEPA) provided editorial, proofreading, and production support; Laurent Bergeron (RBM Partnership Secretariat) assisted with report production; Scott Brown (PATH) assisted with graphic design, Florence Rusciano (WHO) provided considerable support for map development and standardization; and Vincent Becker (Global Fund to Fight AIDS, Tuberculosis and Malaria [GFATM]) gave access to a wide range of photos.

The RBM Progress & Impact Series Oversight Committee members are: Alexandra Farnum (chair), Suprotik Basu, Valentina Buj, John Paul Clark, Alan Court, Alexandra Fullem, Lisa Goldman, Bremen Leak, Eric Mouzin, Robert Newman, and Richard Steketee.

The report's development and production was funded in part by a grant from the Bill & Melinda Gates Foundation to PATH.

The authors are responsible for any errors and omissions.

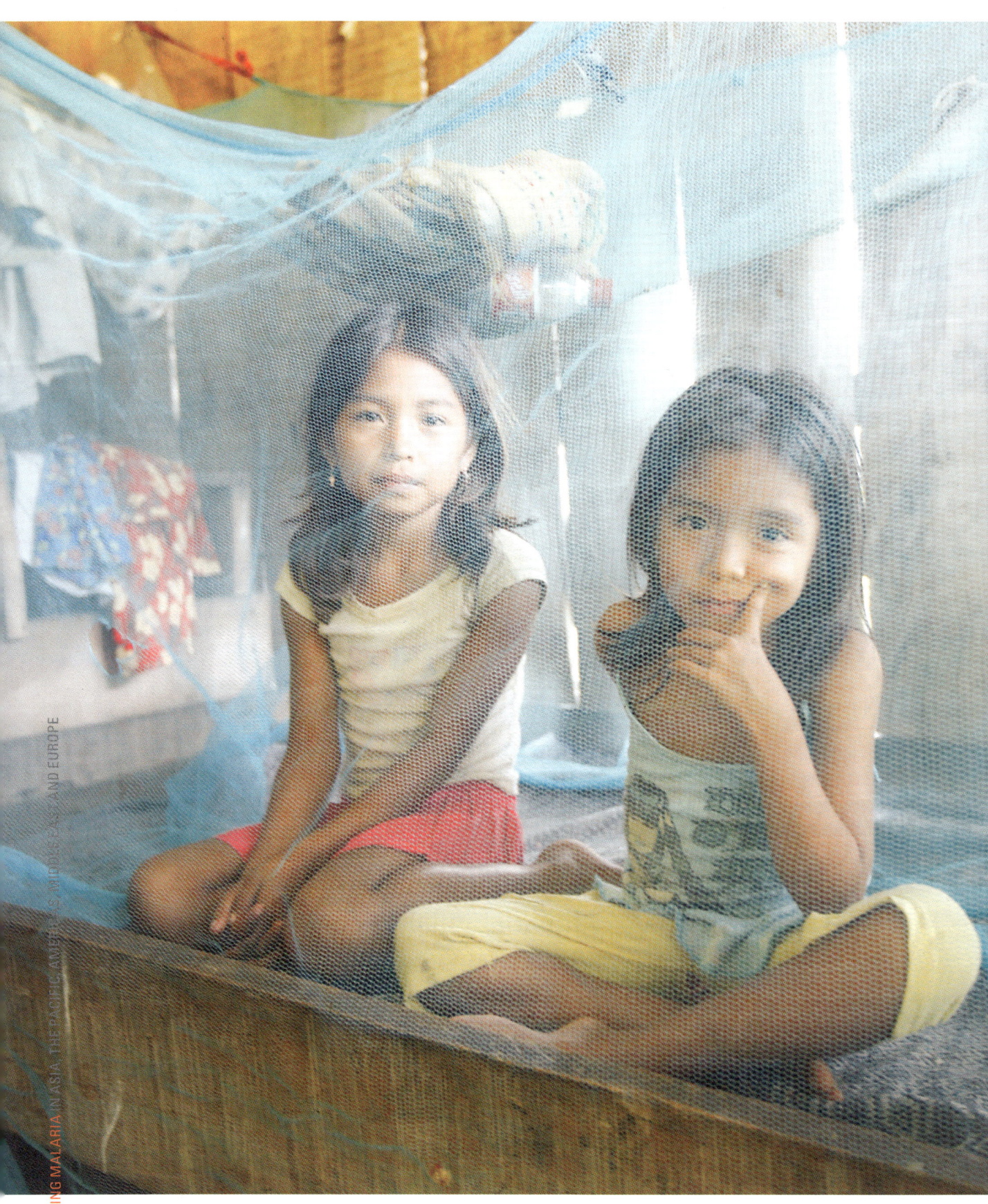

EXECUTIVE SUMMARY

In recent years, the expansion of malaria prevention tools and a scale-up of diagnostic testing and treatment has led to significant progress against the disease in countries outside of Africa. Yet, this mosquito-borne disease continues to impose a major burden on national health systems, requiring tailored control strategies for different geographical areas within countries. The 51 malaria-endemic countries outside of Africa had an estimated 34 million malaria cases in 2010 and approximately 46 000 related deaths.[a] This report focuses on countries in Asia, the Pacific, Americas, Middle East, and Europe because of their unique circumstance; many countries are on the brink of eliminating malaria while at the same time facing challenges that aren't seen elsewhere in the malaria-endemic world.

The level of malaria risk in these regions can vary enormously. It can be as high as in parts of sub-Saharan Africa, with cases and deaths concentrated in children under five years of age, or 1000-fold lower where cases and deaths occur according to the degree of exposure. Malaria's main victims tend to be poorer populations living in rural communities, with limited or no access to long-lasting insecticidal nets (LLINs) and artemisinin-based combination therapies (ACTs). Despite being entirely preventable and treatable, malaria exacts a tragic human toll on societies while its economic and social impact is also devastating. Not only is it disproportionately concentrated in poor and vulnerable communities, it has been a major barrier to economic development, tourism, and foreign investment.

While the disease burden has been declining in countries with fewer malaria cases and deaths, progress has been slower in countries where the bulk of the disease burden lies: India, Indonesia, Myanmar, Pakistan, and Papua New Guinea. These five high-burden countries account for 89% of all malaria cases in the region and need substantial financial resources and technical assistance to strengthen their health systems before they can visibly improve their malaria response. At their current pace, it is unlikely that these countries can achieve the malaria-specific Millennium Development Goals and the World Health Assembly target of reducing the malaria burden by at least 75% by 2015.

The fight against malaria is further complicated by growing parasite resistance to antimalarial drugs. In recent years, artemisinin resistance in the Greater Mekong subregion has become a major and urgent concern. There is a limited window of opportunity to contain resistant parasites before they spread around the world. To avert a regional public health disaster with

[a] The uncertainty range for malaria cases outside of Africa is 32 to 45 million, while for malaria deaths it is 42 000 to 70 000.

| EXECUTIVE SUMMARY |

severe global consequences, containment efforts need to be strengthened while monitoring for the first signs of artemisinin resistance should be intensified in all other endemic countries. In parallel, a coordinated response is needed to tackle emerging insecticide resistance, which—if it goes unchecked—could unravel recent gains both in malaria control and drug resistance containment.

The technical know-how to address challenges and extend progress is available. Technical partners have been working closely with ministries of health on the design, evaluation, and updating of national malaria control strategies and roadmaps. The WHO and the Roll Back Malaria (RBM) Partnership have made available global strategies to tackle both drug and insecticide resistance. The *Global Plan for Artemisinin Resistance Containment* was released in January 2011, while the *Global Plan for Insecticide Resistance Management* was issued in May 2012. WHO also launched the *T3: Test. Treat. Track* initiative in April 2012 to urge countries to scale up diagnostic testing, treatment, and surveillance for malaria.

Established in 1998 by WHO, UNICEF, the United Nations Development Programme, and the World Bank, RBM serves as the overall umbrella for coordinating global malaria control efforts, aligning partners from malaria-endemic countries, multilateral development organizations, the private sector, nongovernmental organizations (NGOs), foundations, and research and academia behind a common strategy to end malaria deaths. The RBM Global Malaria Action Plan, launched in 2008, provides a global framework for action, facilitating collaboration and coordination among different partners. During the past decade, the RBM partnership has built political commitment, improved endemic countries' access to adequate funding, and ensured that WHO policies and recommendations for prevention, diagnosis and treatment of malaria are widely disseminated.

While international funding for malaria control outside of Africa has risen steeply in the last decade, from less than US$ 17 million in 2000 to US$ 300 million in 2010, the amount committed still falls short of the resources required to achieve universal access to life-saving malaria prevention and control measures, estimated at about US$ 3 billion per year. Continued support is necessary to protect current achievements, while greater resources are needed to tackle malaria in areas where it remains most entrenched. Malaria-endemic countries in Asia, the Pacific, Americas, Middle East, and Europe have experienced rapid economic growth between 2000 and 2010, and governments have increased domestic revenues and spending as a consequence. As international funding for malaria control becomes increasingly constrained, endemic countries need to ensure that sufficient domestic resources are allocated for effective malaria control. Without these resources, existing gaps in programme provision cannot be filled and the loftier ambitions of malaria elimination and ultimate eradication cannot be reached.

The effectiveness of the malaria response will continue to depend on the availability of commodities and logistics support provided through key malaria partners such as the Global Fund to Fight AIDS, Tuberculosis and Malaria, as well as UN agencies, donors, and nongovernmental organizations. Firm supply chain management, the prevention of medicine stock-outs, the roll-out of rapid diagnostic tests, and the timely replacement of expired LLINs will also be key to success. Also fundamental are the efforts of the research community and industry partners to advance innovations and scientific breakthroughs that will facilitate the scaling up of interventions and the tackling of drug and insecticide resistance.

With malaria designated as one of the key priorities on the UN Secretary General's five-year action agenda (2012–2017), there is an unprecedented opportunity to end the unnecessary suffering caused by this disease. There is an urgent need to reduce malaria incidence in high-burden countries, and to help countries close to elimination to cross the finish line. Four countries in regions outside of Africa have been certified free of malaria since 2007. Another 17 are in the pre-elimination or elimination stage of malaria control and poised to eliminate malaria, removing the threat of disease from 74 million people currently at risk. Achieving elimination in additional countries outside of Africa would represent a historic achievement, setting the course for eventual eradication of the disease, and providing much-needed impetus to countries in Africa, where the disease is most endemic.

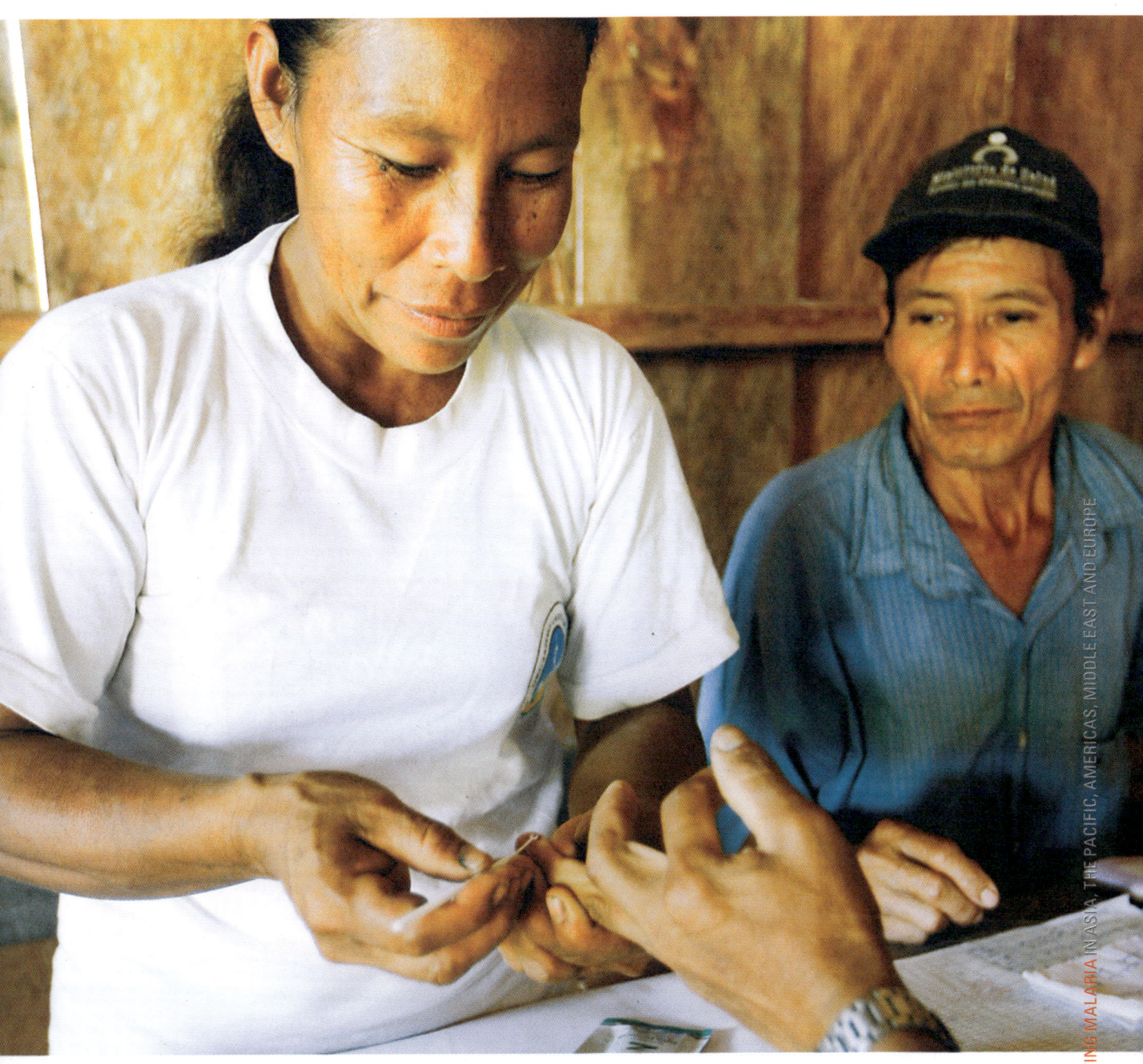

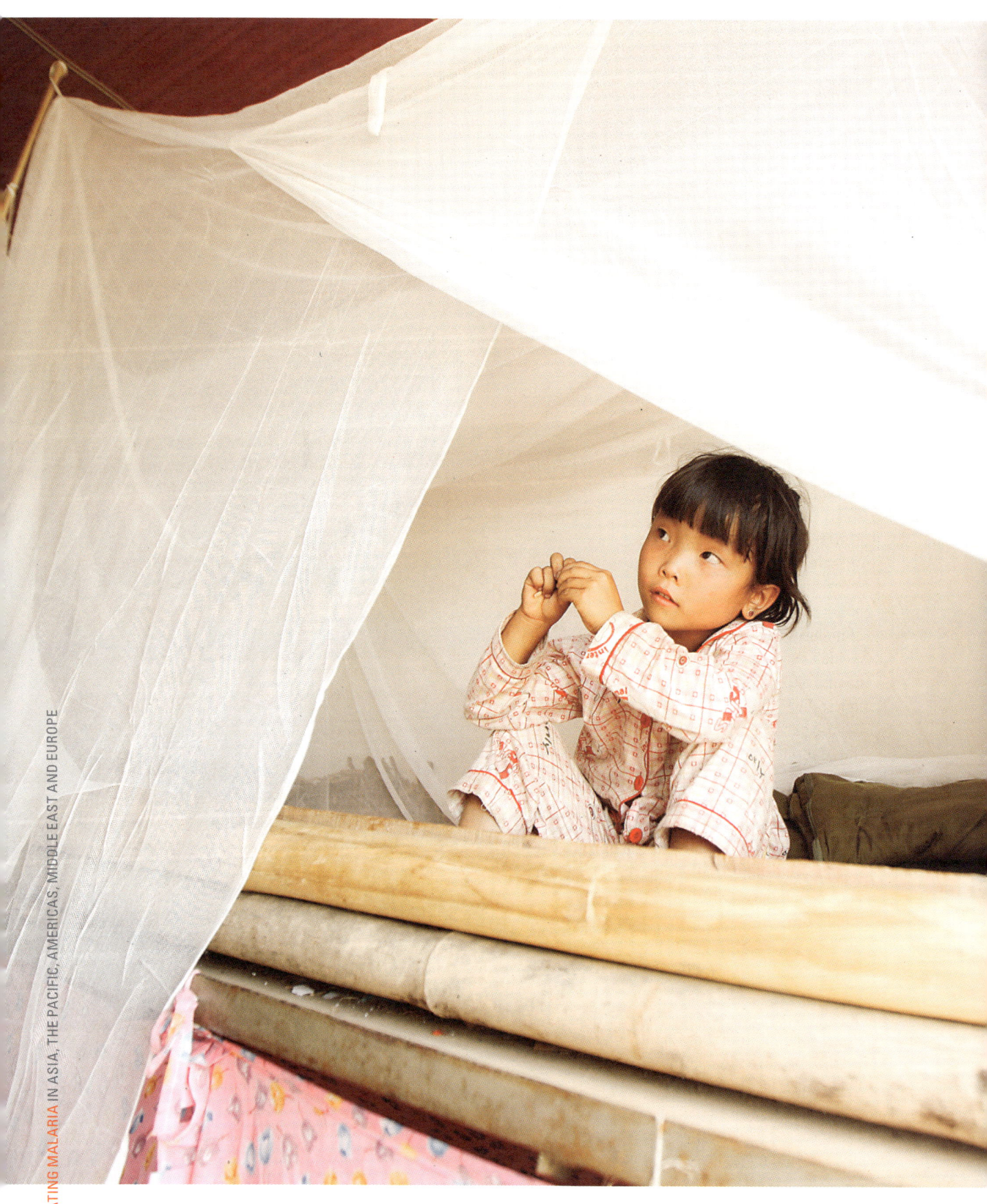

DEFEATING MALARIA IN ASIA, THE PACIFIC, AMERICAS, MIDDLE EAST AND EUROPE

KEY POINTS

1. Malaria remains a public health problem in 51 countries outside of Africa, particularly affecting poorer populations.

- **Malaria remains a public health problem outside of Africa.** It leads to an estimated 34 million cases and 46 000 deaths among a population at risk of 2.5 billion people. The level of malaria risk can vary enormously. It can be as high as in parts of sub-Saharan Africa, with cases and deaths concentrated in children under five years of age, or 1000-fold lower where cases and deaths occur according to the degree of exposure. Both *Plasmodium falciparum* and *P. vivax* parasites occur in great frequency. Diagnostic testing to determine the specific parasite and using the appropriate drug are critical. Malaria outside Africa is also characterized by greater mosquito vector diversity. Different vectors may have widely different breeding, feeding, and resting behaviours. Vector control interventions need to adapt to specific vector characteristics in a locality.

- **Poorer populations are more likely to be affected.** Poorer populations are more likely to live in rural areas in housing that offers little protection against mosquitoes. Furthermore, they are less likely to have access to mosquito nets or indoor residual spraying (IRS). They also tend to live further away from health facilities that can offer effective diagnostic testing and treatment and be less able to afford quality treatment.

- **Malaria imposes costs on society which go beyond the costs to individuals and families affected by the disease.** Productivity of businesses and government is reduced because of employee work time lost due to illness, and extra costs are incurred in preventing, diagnosing, and treating malaria. Malaria can discourage investment and trade—markets may be undeveloped owing to traders' unwillingness to travel to and invest in malaria-endemic areas. A country's tourist industry may remain undeveloped due to the travelers' reluctance to visiting malaria-endemic areas.

2. Progress in defeating malaria has been substantial.

- **Funding for malaria control has increased.** Since 2003, international funding for malaria control has risen by more than eight-fold primarily because of the growth in funding from the Global Fund to Fight AIDS, Tuberculosis and Malaria, which accounted for approximately 88% of the US$ 300 million of international funds disbursed for malaria control outside of

| KEY POINTS |

Africa in 2010. A further 8% of international funding was from the World Bank and another 2% from the Australian government. The growth in international funding for malaria control has been matched, in some instances, by increases in domestic spending.

- **Malaria control programmes have been expanded.** The increased funding has enabled worldwide implementation of malaria control interventions, including long-lasting insecticidal mosquito nets (LLINs) and IRS for the prevention of malaria, and rapid diagnostic tests (RDTs) and ACTs for the diagnosis and treatment of malaria. The large-scale implementation of interventions against malaria has led to widespread reductions in malaria cases and deaths and a shrinking of areas affected by malaria.

- **The number of malaria cases and deaths has decreased.** A total of 34 countries outside of Africa have reduced cases by more than 50% since 2000. Malaria death rates have decreased by 30% outside of Africa and four countries have been certified as free of malaria since 2007 (Armenia, Morocco, Turkmenistan, and the United Arab Emirates). The World Health Organization (WHO) European Region is aiming for elimination of malaria across the entire region by 2015 and *P. falciparum* transmission has already been eliminated from the region. Another 17 countries are in the pre-elimination or elimination phases of malaria control and on the brink of eliminating malaria from within their boundaries.

3. Further progress is possible but major challenges lie ahead.

- **Mechanisms for the delivery of malaria interventions have been developed.** In most countries outside of Africa, delivery mechanisms have been established for mass distribution of LLINs and ensuring access to diagnostic testing and treatment in remote communities. Partnerships among different organizations involved in malaria control have, under the Roll back Malaria (RBM) umbrella, been established, to gain economies of scale and ensure that WHO policies for prevention, diagnosis, and treatment of malaria are disseminated to implementing partners and activities are coordinated to ensure a more rational allocation of resources.

- **Progress has been substantial in countries with fewer malaria cases and deaths but slower in countries where the bulk of the disease burden lies.** The 34 countries that halved their malaria case numbers between 2000 and 2010 accounted for only 14% of all non-African cases in 2000 (8.3 million cases out of 59 million estimated). Greater attention is needed to reducing the burden of malaria in countries where the problem is greatest.

- **As malaria decreases it is increasingly concentrated in marginalized populations.** Ethnic, religious, and political minorities are particularly affected as are migrant workers and populations living in less developed border regions. It is more challenging, and more costly, to offer services to these populations because of geographical accessibility, security, or political concerns.

- **As malaria decreases, *P. vivax* malaria—which is more difficult to control—becomes more prominent.** As malaria control is intensified, the number of cases due to *P. falciparum* falls more quickly than those of *P. vivax* so the proportion of cases due to *P. vivax* increases. Although *P. vivax* infections are less likely to lead to severe malaria and death it is more difficult to control because it has a dormant liver stage which cannot be detected with existing diagnostic tests and can only be eliminated by administering primaquine which must be taken daily over 14 days. Primaquine can produce serious side-effects (hemolytic anaemia) in patients who have more severe forms of glucose-6-phosphate dehydrogenase (G6PD) deficiency. The development of a low-cost and accurate RDT for G6PD deficiency would be an important advance for the control of *vivax* malaria.

- **As disease incidence decreases populations are more prone to epidemics.** As the incidence of malaria is reduced, naturally acquired immunity to the disease (which is at best partial) decreases. Although new infections are less likely to occur they can rapidly lead to illness, which can be severe, and they can more easily spread from one person to another. A high level of commitment is needed to maintain control programmes even once success has been achieved.

- **Unique diversity in behaviour of the mosquito vectors presents additional challenges.** These mosquitoes are diverse in their biting and resting habits and their living and breeding habitats. For example, some efficient vectors live and breed in forested regions and bite and rest outdoors and are therefore not easily controlled by insecticide-treated mosquito nets or IRS.

- **Resistance to the latest antimalarial medicines has emerged in South-East Asia.** *P. falciparum* resistance to artemisinins has been detected in Cambodia, Myanmar, Thailand, and Viet Nam. Although the large majority of patients with delayed response to artemisinins are currently still being cured when treated with an ACT, resistance needs to be contained in existing hotspots before it is spread around the world and the ability to treat *P. falciparum* malaria is lost worldwide. No other antimalarial medicines are available at present with the same level of efficacy and tolerability as ACTs, and the earliest that replacement medicines could be available is 2016.

- **Resistance to the insecticides used to control mosquitoes is widespread.** Existing vector control tools are currently effective in the vast majority of settings. However, insecticide resistance has now been reported in 24 out of 51 countries with malaria transmission outside of Africa. Resistance to a class of chemicals known as pyrethroids, which are the most commonly used chemicals for IRS and the only class used on LLINs, seems most widespread. Resistance to these chemicals could severely impact the ability to maintain gains already achieved in reducing malaria as well as the ability to aim for further success.

- **Future funding for malaria control in Asia, the Pacific, Americas, Middle East, and Europe is threatened.** Many endemic countries are particularly reliant on the Global Fund, which accounts for the vast majority of international disbursements for malaria control. The Global Fund has recently experienced lower levels of replenishment than expected and Round 11 of the Global Fund's application process was cancelled to be replaced with a transitional funding mechanism which aims to sustain existing investments. Along with other donors, the Global Fund is increasingly focusing its funding on the poorest countries in Africa with the highest malaria burden. International funding for countries outside of Africa may therefore decrease.

4. What needs to be done?

To achieve the ambitious global goals of reducing the needless loss of life due to malaria, and to further reduce the malaria burden outside of Africa, governments, development partners, and other stakeholders should focus their attention on six priority areas.

1. Bridge the funding gap. While more money is available for malaria control outside of Africa than ever before, these resources still fall short of the amount required for effective disease control.

| KEY POINTS |

An unprecedented global fundraising effort is needed—mobilizing both existing and emerging donors—to ensure that all endemic countries move closer to elimination, marginalized populations are reached, and the efforts to contain drug and insecticide resistance are scaled up. It will also be critical that malaria-endemic countries benefiting from economic growth allocate more domestic resources to fight malaria, or the progress made in reducing malaria to date will be put at risk.

2. Increase technical assistance and knowledge transfers. To defeat malaria, many endemic countries will also need significantly more technical assistance to strengthen their malaria response. When requested, technical partners should scale up assistance to ministries of health to support them in their efforts to design, evaluate, and update national malaria control strategies and work plans. Development partners should continue to help ministries of health provide health worker training and strengthen human resources for health. Particular attention should be paid to the design of interventions that help vulnerable groups be reached.

3. Provide universal access to preventive interventions. Greater efforts are needed to provide protection to all those at risk of malaria, particularly in the most populous countries with the greatest numbers of cases and deaths. Attainment of this goal will be particularly challenging for those communities that are mobile or live in remote border areas. In some situations, novel vector control methods may be needed, such as insecticide-treated hammocks to protect those who work and sleep in forests overnight, or insecticidal mosquito coils to protect against outdoor biting mosquitoes. As prevalence rates fall and remain very low in many areas, new approaches need to be developed to tackle the last remaining cases.

4. Scale up diagnostic testing, treatment, and surveillance. With the 2012 launch of WHO's *T3: Test. Treat. Track* initiative, malaria-endemic countries and donors are urged to ensure that every suspected malaria case is tested, that every confirmed case is treated with a quality-assured antimalarial medicine, and that the disease is tracked through timely and accurate surveillance systems. Scaling up these three interconnected pillars will provide the much-needed bridge between efforts to achieve universal coverage with prevention tools and the goal of eliminating malaria. It will also lead to a better overall understanding of the distribution of the disease, and enable national malaria control programmes to most efficiently direct available resources to where they are needed. T3 scale-up will enable affected countries to deliver a better return on investment on malaria funding received from international donors.

5. Step up the fight against drug and insecticide resistance. The double threat of drug and insecticide resistance imperils recent gains in malaria prevention and control. Increased political commitment and new sources of funding will be needed to tackle these challenges. WHO has made global strategies available to address both drug and insecticide resistance. The *Global Plan for Artemisinin Resistance Containment* was released in January 2011, while the *Global Plan for Insecticide Resistance Management in malaria vectors* was issued in May 2012. These plans should be fully implemented by governments and stakeholders in the global malaria community to preserve the current tools of malaria control until new and more effective tools become available. Contributions from the research community and industry partners will be fundamental to tackling these emerging threats.

6. Strengthen regional cooperation. Malaria can be defeated only if governments scale up regional cooperation efforts to strengthen the regulatory environment for pharmaceuticals and work together on removing oral artemisinin-based monotherapies and counterfeit medicines from markets. Countries also need to collaborate on managing the supply chain for malaria commodities and share information about drug and insecticide resistance patterns. In a world where malaria is increasingly confined to border areas—and where cross-border migration represents a major source of new malaria infection—regional cooperation is also critical for the development of cross-border strategies that are inclusive of marginalized populations.

Governments have already made a number of commitments in the UN General Assembly and the World Health Assembly, through the governing bodies of WHO regional structures,[b] and through a range of regional cooperation platforms, such as the Union of South American Nations (UNASUR) and the Association of Southeast Asian Nations (ASEAN). However, stronger political commitment will be needed to provide universal access to all key malaria interventions and to move closer to malaria elimination. With malaria designated as one of the key priorities of the UN Secretary General's five-year action agenda (2012–2017), there is an unprecedented opportunity to end the unnecessary suffering caused by this disease.

5. What can be gained?

- **The burden of a senseless, preventable tragedy can be lifted.** Scaling up malaria control efforts has been proven to reduce illness and death, especially among the poorest populations outside of Africa. This relieves some of the most vulnerable populations of a significant illness that causes disruption to schooling, work, and, at the worst, death.

- **Considerable long-term impact and financial savings can be achieved both in endemic countries and globally.** Protecting the tools we have by working to contain emerging drug and insecticide resistance will have cost implications in the near term for which many malaria-endemic countries will need support. However, investment now will result in significant savings in the long run, improving the sustainability and public health impact of malaria interventions, not only in countries affected but globally.

- **Health systems can be strengthened.** Improving the malaria response—at both the national level and in larger regions—will boost the capacities of health systems to improve the treatment of other febrile illnesses and will help to direct financial resources where the funds are most needed. Strengthening health infrastructure and improving health information systems for malaria will strengthen countries' overall capacities to respond to future public health threats, while also helping bridge existing health inequalities.

- **Large areas of the world can be free of malaria in the foreseeable future.** Four countries outside of Africa have been certified free of malaria since 2007. Another 17 are in the pre-elimination or elimination stage of malaria control and poised to eliminate malaria soon—removing the threat of disease from 74 million people currently at risk. If elimination is attained in these countries it would represent a historic achievement to be remembered for decades to come and set the course for eventual eradication of this ancient disease.

---

[b] See, for instance, the Regional Action Plan for Malaria Control and Elimination in the Western Pacific (2010–2015), which was endorsed by the 60th Regional Committee of the WHO Western Pacific Region in 2009.

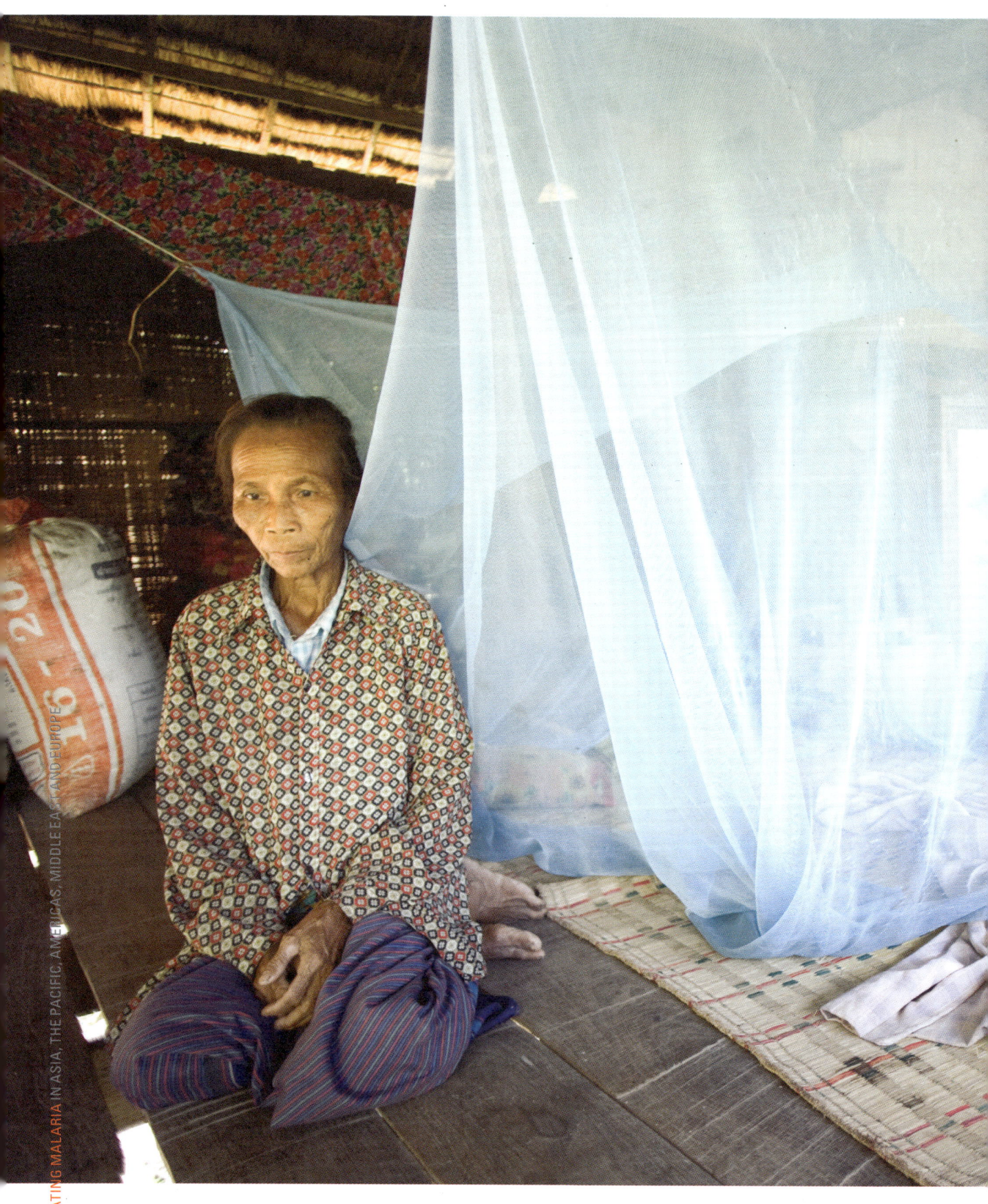

CHAPTER I

INTRODUCTION: MALARIA OUTSIDE OF AFRICA IS A DISEASE OF POVERTY THAT POSES UNIQUE CHALLENGES FOR CONTROL

Malaria exacts a heavy toll in Asia, the Pacific, Americas, Middle East, and Europe. While the disease burden is heaviest in Africa, outside of Africa there are 51 countries where malaria is a very real public health problem that threatens many, especially the poor and marginalized. The disease negatively affects family income due to lost income and payment for treatment. It affects business due to direct costs of lost production, absenteeism, and prevention and treatment. The biology of the parasite, the mosquito vectors, and the human population at risk are considerably more diverse outside Africa, thus presenting a range of unique challenges.

While Africa is widely understood to carry the major burden of malaria, the disease constitutes a significant public health problem in 51 countries elsewhere in the world where it is inextricably linked with poverty (Figure 1.1).

Poorer populations are more likely to be exposed to malaria-carrying mosquitoes because they are more likely to live in rural areas in housing that offers little protection against mosquitoes and they are less likely to have access to mosquito nets or indoor residual spraying of insecticides (IRS). They also tend to live further away from health facilities that can offer effective diagnostic testing and treatment and to be less able to afford quality treatment.

An episode of malaria reduces the days worked not only of the infected but of those that care for them. The Indian Commission on Macroeconomics and Health notes that, in India, 13 household person-days per patient were lost per episode of malaria. Furthermore, the commission estimated that the overall monetary losses to families (income losses together with treatment expenses) could amount to between 200 and 400 Indian rupees (US$ 3.5 to 7) (*1*). The poorest 10% of the Indian population rely on sales of their assets or on borrowing to pay for health-care services, reducing a family's ability to access basic goods and affecting their long-term economic prospects.

| INTRODUCTION |

Figure 1.1
Malaria and poverty
Countries with higher proportions of their population living in poverty (less than US$ 1.25 per day) have higher death rates from malaria.

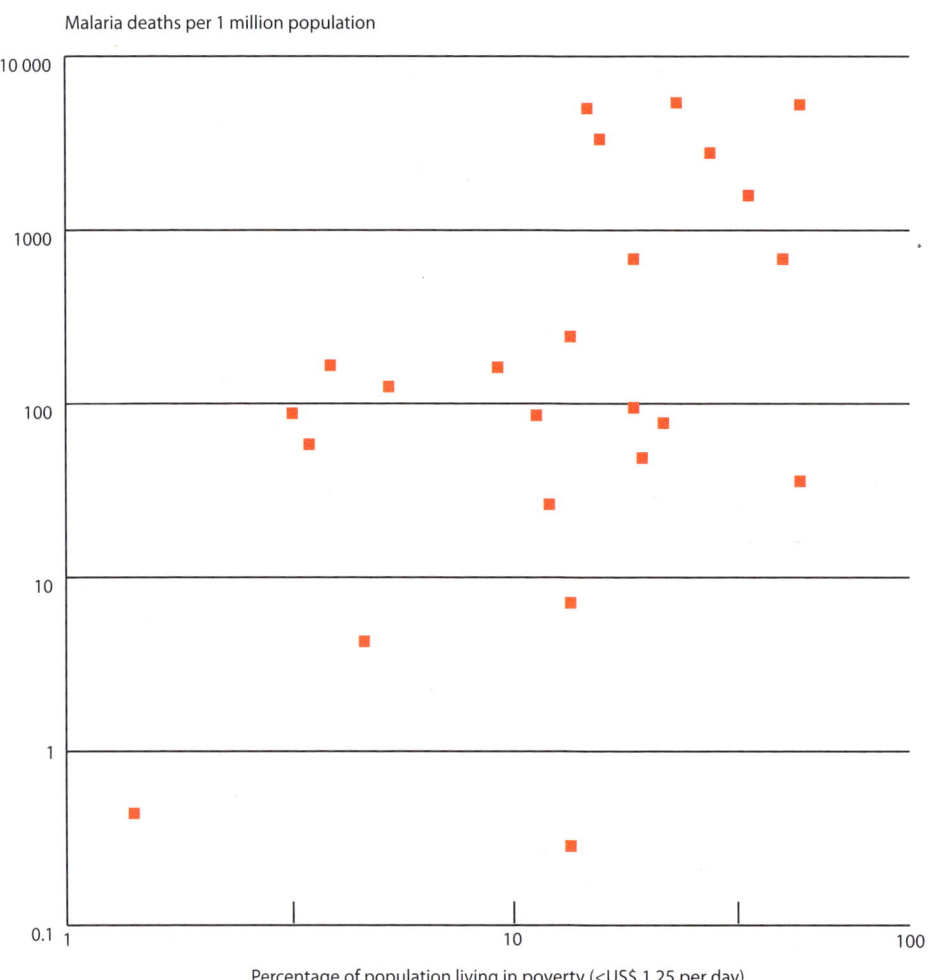

Note: This illustrative figure shows the poverty and malaria mortality rates for 24 malaria-endemic countries outside of Africa.
Source of poverty data: Human Development Report 2011.
Source of malaria mortality rates: World Malaria Report 2011.

Malaria imposes costs on society which extend beyond the costs to individuals and families affected by the disease. With an estimated 22.5 million malaria cases in India (2), this translates to an annual cost of US$ 79 to 157 million, or 0.01% of gross domestic product each year.[c] In states with the highest incidence rates, such as Chhattisgarh, Jharkhand, Meghalaya, Mizoram, and Orissa, the annual cost of illness represents more than 0.1% of a gross state income.

Businesses and governments lose production and incur extra costs in preventing, diagnosing, and treating malaria. In Higaturu Oil Palm plantation, Papua New Guinea, 2015 malaria cases were diagnosed among employees in 2006. On average, an employee sick with malaria was absent for 1.8 days per episode resulting in more than 3600 workdays lost in 2006 (3).

Malaria can also discourage investment and trade—markets may be undeveloped owing to traders' unwillingness to travel to and invest in malaria-endemic areas. A country's tourist industry may remain undeveloped due to reluctance of travelers to visit malaria-endemic areas. This further limits economic growth in some of the poorest regions of the world.

While malaria transmission in Asia, the Pacific, Americas, Middle East, and Europe is generally less intense than in Africa there are unique challenges for control. The biology of the parasite, the mosquito vectors, and the human population at risk are considerably more diverse. The distribution of malaria parasites is heterogeneous and approximately half of infections are due to *P. vivax* rather than *P. falciparum*, requiring prolonged treatment with primaquine to eliminate liver stages and therefore prevent later relapses. The mosquito vectors of malaria are also diverse in their biting and resting habits and their living and breeding habitats. Vector control is more challenging in some areas because of this diversity. For example, some efficient vectors live and breed in forested regions and bite and rest outdoors and are therefore not easily controlled by insecticide-treated mosquito nets (ITNs) or IRS. The populations most affected frequently live in remote areas and/or are marginalized groups such as migrant workers, tribal populations, or those living in border areas.

The risk of malaria infection in populations outside of Africa is also greatly variable. In some settings, such as parts of Papua New Guinea, transmission can be intense and individuals may experience many infections each year, experiencing "Africa-like malaria". In other areas, transmission intensity is so low that even though there may be some risk, less than one person in a thousand will acquire an infection in a given year. In some areas infection rates are so low that little immunity is developed against malaria so that, with certain suitable climate and social conditions, transmission can rapidly increase and cause epidemics if public health control efforts are withdrawn.

The tremendous diversity of situations outside of Africa demands that a broader range of strategies be adopted for malaria control. This report summarizes some of the main features of the epidemiology of malaria outside of Africa, the enormous progress that has been made in controlling malaria, and some of the challenges that remain.

---

[c] The uncertainty range for malaria cases in India is 17 to 30 million.

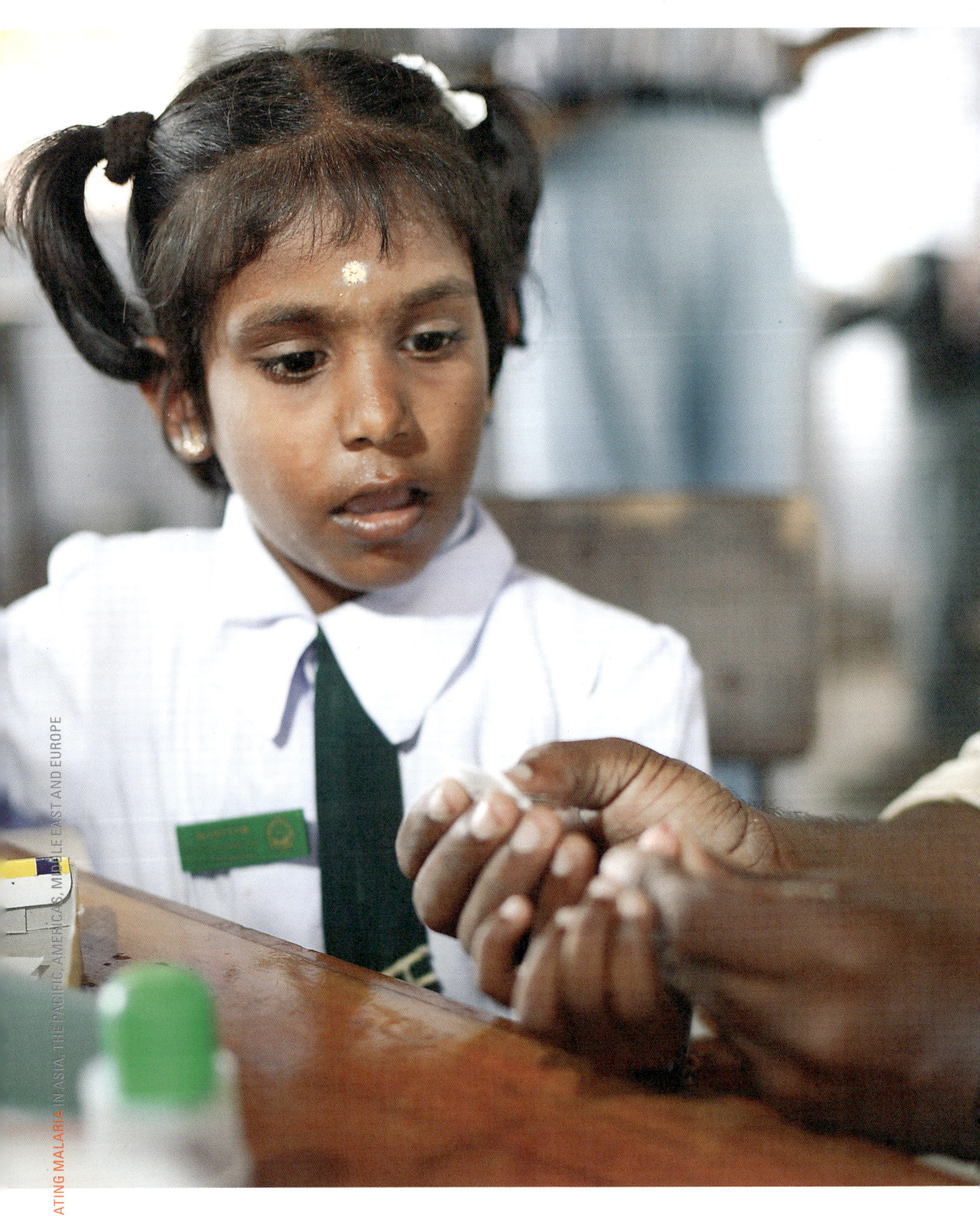

CHAPTER II

GLOBAL OVERVIEW OF MALARIA EPIDEMIOLOGY

Ongoing malaria transmission is present in 99 countries and territories worldwide, about half of which are in Africa. Most of these countries are in the control phase, and the remainder is essentially evenly split between being in pre-elimination, elimination, and prevention of reintroduction phases. Of the five Plasmodium *parasites that infect humans (P. falciparum, P. vivax, P. ovale, P. malariae, and* P. knowlesi*),* P. falciparum *causes the most deaths and* P. vivax *causes much illness but few deaths. An estimated 216 million malaria cases and 655 000 deaths occurred globally in 2010; 16% of those cases occurred outside of Africa, more than half which were attributable to* P. falciparum. *Treatments of the two parasite types differ, making accurate diagnostics important in areas where both species are present. The* P. vivax *parasite can develop in the mosquito vector at lower temperatures and survive at higher altitudes than can* P. falciparum. P. vivax *can remain dormant in the liver for long periods, where it is impossible to diagnose. The female Anopheles mosquito spreads malaria from person to person, and the* Anopheles *species responsible for malaria transmission in Africa differs in type, behaviour and characteristics from that which is responsible outside of that region. These differences have important implications on which methods of vector control (ITNs and IRS) are used, and how.*

Countries with malaria transmission

There are 99 countries and territories with ongoing transmission of malaria. Of these, 48 lie on the African continent, 21 are in the Americas, and 30 in Europe, Asia, and the Pacific. Of the 99 countries and territories, 82 are in the control phase, 8 in the pre-elimination phase, and 9 in the elimination phase (see Map 2.1). A further 8 countries are in the prevention of reintroduction phase.

Map 2.1
Phases of malaria control among all malaria-endemic countries, 2011

Malaria-endemic countries are classified into one of four categories (control, pre-elimination, elimination, or prevention of reintroduction), depending on the phase of their programme.

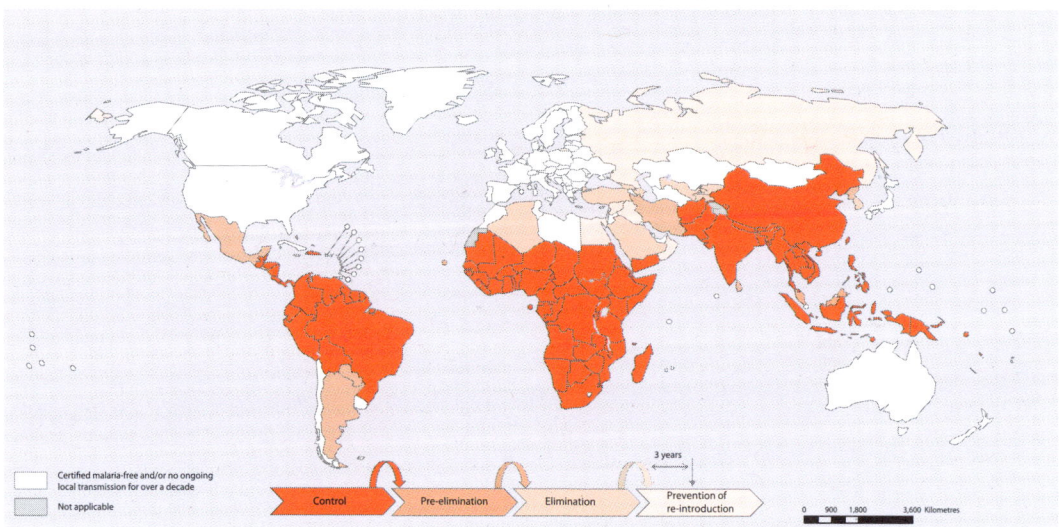

Source: World Health Organization, 2011.
Map production: WHO Global Malaria Programme.

Types of malaria

Malaria is caused by infection with the human parasite *Plasmodium*. There are five species that infect humans: *Plasmodium falciparum*, *P. vivax*, *P. ovale*, *P. malariae*, and *P. knowlesi*. Of these, the first two are the most important. *P. falciparum* is the most deadly while *P. vivax* causes much illness but few deaths (Box 2.1). Uncomplicated *P. falciparum* malaria is treated with an artemisinin-based combination therapy (ACT) while *P. vivax* malaria is treated with chloroquine in areas where it remains effective,[d] together with primaquine in order to prevent relapses. In areas where the two species occur together it is important to know which species is responsible for an infection so the appropriate treatment course can be selected. This requires that all suspected malaria cases are given a parasitological test by microscopy or malaria rapid diagnostic test (RDT) to confirm the illness is due to *Plasmodium* and to determine the species of parasite[e] (Box 2.2).

---

[d] *P. vivax* should be treated with an appropriate ACT rather than chloroquine in areas where *P. vivax* resistance to chloroquine has been documented.
[e] Some RDTs are only able to detect *P. falciparum*. Positive cases are therefore given an ACT while negative cases may be treated as *P. vivax*.

Box 2.1: Comparison of *P. falciparum* and *P. vivax* malaria

Life cycle	*P. falciparum*	*P. vivax*
Minimum temperature needed for maturation in the mosquito	Lowest temperature 16 °C (*4*)	For cycle to be complete lowest temperature 15 °C, survival of parasite to 10 °C for two days (*5*)
Dormant liver stage	No	Yes
Gametocytes	Appear after asexual blood stage is established	Appear at time of asexual blood stage often before clinical symptoms
Disease		
Severity	5% of cases develop into severe illness	< 1% develop into severe illness
Relapse possible	No	Yes
Asymptomatic carriage	Common	Very common
Diagnosis		
Blood stage	Blood film, rapid tests and PCR for blood stage	Blood film, rapid tests and PCR for blood stage
Liver stage		No test for dormant liver stage
Treatment		
Blood stage	Artemisinin combination treatment (ACT) recommended	Chloroquine still efficacious in most areas
Gametocytes	Need single dose primaquine, artemesinins have some effect	Sensitive to blood stage treatment
Liver stage		14 days of primaquine

Box 2.2: Diagnosing *P. falciparum* and *P. vivax*

A brief summary of approaches to malaria diagnostic testing is provided below. More detailed information can be found in *Universal access to malaria diagnostic testing: an operational manual* (*4*) and the other documents cited below.

Microscopy: Light microscopy has been the standard for malaria diagnosis for many decades and is still the primary method of malaria diagnosis in health clinics and hospitals throughout the world. It is the only widespread method of differentiating between all major *Plasmodium species*, *P. falciparum*, *P. vivax*, *P. malariae*, and *P. ovale*, as well as for detecting gametocytes of *P. falciparum* and mixed infections. Microscopy can provide parasite counts (i.e. estimates of parasite density in peripheral blood) and can therefore be used to monitor response to treatment. Microscopy requires functioning equipment, regular provision of laboratory supplies, well-trained laboratory technicians at all levels, regular supervision, and a functional quality management system. For this reason, it is generally more widely available in countries with more resources and more robust health systems.

The sensitivity and specificity of light microscopy are directly related to the time available to read a blood film, the quality of the stained film, and the competence of the microscopist. Good microscopists in health facilities can detect as few as 100–200 parasites per microlitre and expert microscopists can detect 50 parasites per microlitre. In most endemic areas, nearly all clinical illness truly due to malaria is thought to correspond to > 100 parasites per microlitre; therefore, a good microscopist should detect parasites in nearly all true clinical malaria cases (*5*). Occasionally, clinical cases may occur at lower parasite densities, particularly very early in the course of an infection.

WHO has suggested competence levels for microscopists, with those at the expert level expected to achieve 90% detection, 90% correct species identification and a high level of quantification (to be within 25% of the true value 90% of the time), and acceptable levels of clinical competence below this value (*6*). In low-transmission settings, high specificity is vital but is hard to maintain. Field microscopy standards are often low, and rigorous quality management systems are necessary to maintain sufficient performance for both malaria case management and surveillance.

Rapid diagnostic tests: In areas where microscopy is not available, especially in high-burden countries, RDTs are becoming increasingly available as the standard for malaria testing in outpatient settings. Several RDTs currently on the market can consistently detect over 95% of parasite infections at 200 parasites per microlitre, with 95% specificity. The three main groups of antigens detected by RDTs are:

- Histidine-rich protein 2, which is specific to *P. falciparum*.

- *Plasmodium* lactate dehydrogenase (pLDH), currently used in products that include *P. falciparum*-specific (pLDH-Pf), pan-specific (pLDH-Pan) antibodies present in all human malaria species, and *P. vivax*-specific pLDH (pLDH-Pv) and non-*falciparum*-specific (pLDH-vom) antibodies.

- Aldolase, which is pan-specific.

Different products on the market have different combinations of antibodies that can detect the above antigens. RDTs that detect both *falciparum*-specific and non-*falciparum* (or pan-specific) target antigens are commonly called "combination" or "combo" tests. The most common formats of RDT products are a plastic cassette and dipsticks; cassettes tend to be simpler to use than dipsticks and have been deployed on a wider scale.

WHO has published the results of RDT performance evaluations against panels of wild-type parasites diluted at specific densities and assessed for stability at high temperatures and ease of use (*7*). The evaluations show wide variation in the performance of different products and procurement should be undertaken in the light of good evidence. An interactive guide designed to help national malaria control programmes select malaria RDTs with specific performance characteristics is available (*8*). Training, supervision, and performance evaluations of health workers using RDTs are also a necessary part of RDT programmes.

Polymerase chain reaction (PCR) tests: The new method of PCR, which is more sensitive than light microscopy or RDTs, is being used for research and field studies for detecting submicroscopic infections, especially with rare species (*P. malariae*, *P. ovale*, and *P. knowlesi*), mixed infections, and low-density infections. In Cambodia, for example, in a national survey in 2007 in which the populations of 76 villages were screened, 13 more villages with malaria cases were identified with PCR than with microscopy (*9*). During screening and treatment in Pailin, Cambodia, in 2008–2009, use of PCR with feedback and treatment of positive cases made it possible to identify and treat 86 asymptomatic carriers (*P. vivax* in most cases) among the 928 people screened, instead of 6 identified and treated when only RDTs were used (*10*).

The relation between the incidence of symptomatic malaria and the prevalence of asymptomatic infections in a population (called the "reservoir") is not fully understood. It depends partly on the prevalence of low-density infections: the lower the overall parasite prevalence in a population, the more additional infections will be found by PCR than by microscopy (*11*). It also depends on the speed at which malaria transmission decreases: when the decrease in transmission is more rapid than loss of immunity in a population the reservoir of asymptomatic carriers can be significant and mass screening is potentially appropriate. For example, in Cambodia microscopy suggested a 3% prevalence rate whereas PCR resulted in a prevalence rate of 7%. When transmission has decreased over many years—for instance in the Brazilian mountains outside of Amazonia where there is a prevalence rate of 0% by microscopy, 0.5% by PCR for *P. falciparum*, and 1.5% by PCR for *P. vivax* (*12*), or in two districts in Sri Lanka with a prevalence rate of 0% by PCR in two districts (*13*)—most people with parasitaemia are symptomatic because they have no immunity and the reservoir is minimal. In these situations mass screening will probably not be cost-effective.

The potential programme value of detecting low-density infections that are microscopy-negative but PCR-positive is unclear.

GLOBAL OVERVIEW OF MALARIA EPIDEMIOLOGY

Geographical distribution

P. vivax has a wider distribution than *P. falciparum* as it is able to develop in the mosquito vector at lower temperatures and survive at higher altitudes and in cooler climates. It also has a dormant liver stage (known as a hypnozoite) which enables it to survive during periods when *Anopheles* mosquitoes are not present to continue transmission, such as during winter months. *P. falciparum* predominates in Africa. Although *P. vivax* can occur throughout Africa, the risk of *P. vivax* infection is considerably reduced in the region by the high frequency of the Duffy negativity trait amongst many African populations; in individuals without the Duffy antigen, red blood cells are resistant to infection with *P. vivax*. In many areas outside of Africa, infections due to *P. vivax* are more common than those due to *P. falciparum* (Map 2.2). A total of 2.37 billion people were considered to be at risk of *P. falciparum* malaria in 2007 of which 1.71 billion lived outside Africa, while 2.85 billion were considered to be at risk of *P. vivax* malaria in 2009 of which 2.75 billion lived outside of Africa (*14*, *15*). However, while some countries report a very large population is at risk, this risk may be very low. For example, China reported 787 million people were at some risk in 2010 but reported less than 8000 cases for an annual risk of 1 infection per 100 000 population-at-risk; taking the high-risk population of 14.3 million and assuming that the infections only occur in this population, it is still an annual risk of less than 1 infection per 1000 population-at-risk.

Disease burden

WHO estimates that 216 million cases of malaria occurred globally in 2010; 34 million (16%) of these occurred outside of Africa of which 18.1 million (53%) were due to *P. falciparum* (Figure 2.1). WHO also estimates that 655 000 deaths occurred globally, of which 46 000 (7%) occurred outside of Africa. WHO estimates that 2.5 billion people were at risk of malaria outside of Africa, thus, while more people are at risk of malaria outside of Africa the number of cases and deaths is much smaller, illustrating that the risk of acquiring malaria outside of Africa is generally lower (*16*).

Vectors

Malaria is spread from one person to another by female mosquitoes of the genus *Anopheles*. There are about 400 different species of *Anopheles* mosquitoes, but only 30 of these are vectors of major importance. The *Anopheles* species responsible for malaria transmission outside of Africa are different to those in Africa. Box 2.3 gives some examples of the different vectors and their behaviour. Some are highly efficient in transmitting malaria and are a particular threat to human populations while others only become important when vector numbers are large. Usually, in any one area there is a dominant vector species that is responsible for most malaria transmission; these are called primary vectors. Vectors of lesser importance are called secondary vectors. Control efforts are usually targeted against the primary vector. The distribution of primary malaria vectors is shown in Map 2.3.

Map 2.2
Proportion of cases due to *P. falciparum*, 2010

In many areas outside of Africa, infections due to P. vivax *are more common than those due to* P. falciparum.

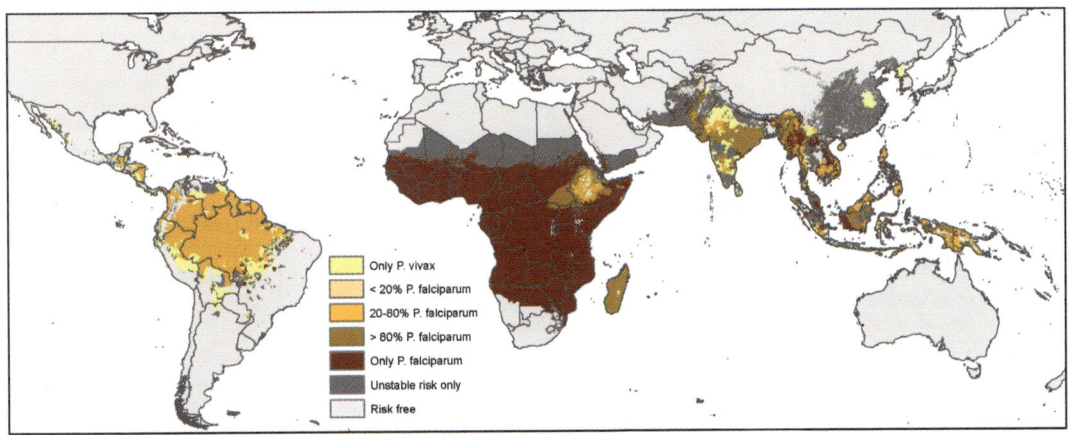

Note: Proportions are based on a four-year average of calculated annual parasite index for *P. falciparum* and *P. vivax* through 2010 and may not reflect the most recently reported subnational data.
Map production and source: Malaria Atlas Project (*17, 18*).

Figure 2.1
Estimated cases of malaria outside of Africa, 2010

WHO estimates that 216 million cases of malaria occurred globally in 2010; 34 million (16%) of these occurred outside of Africa of which 18.1 million (53%) were due to P. falciparum.

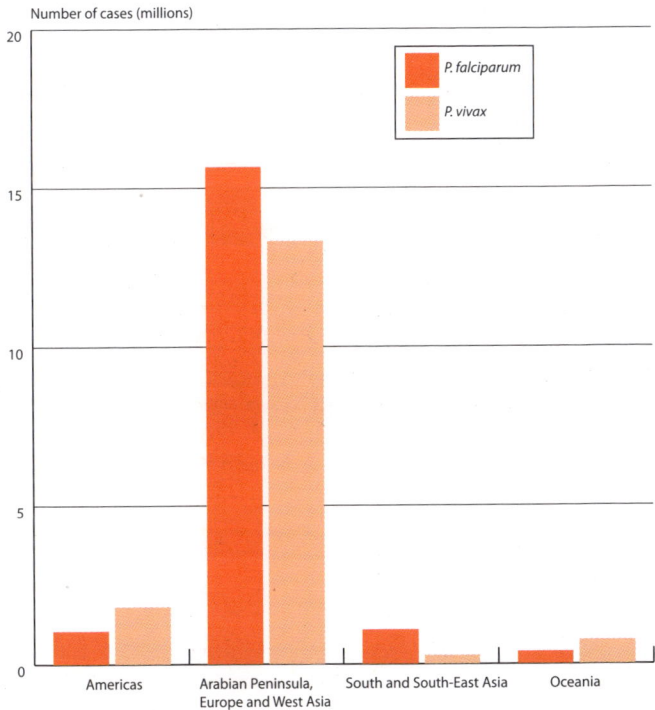

Source: World Malaria Report 2011 (*16*).

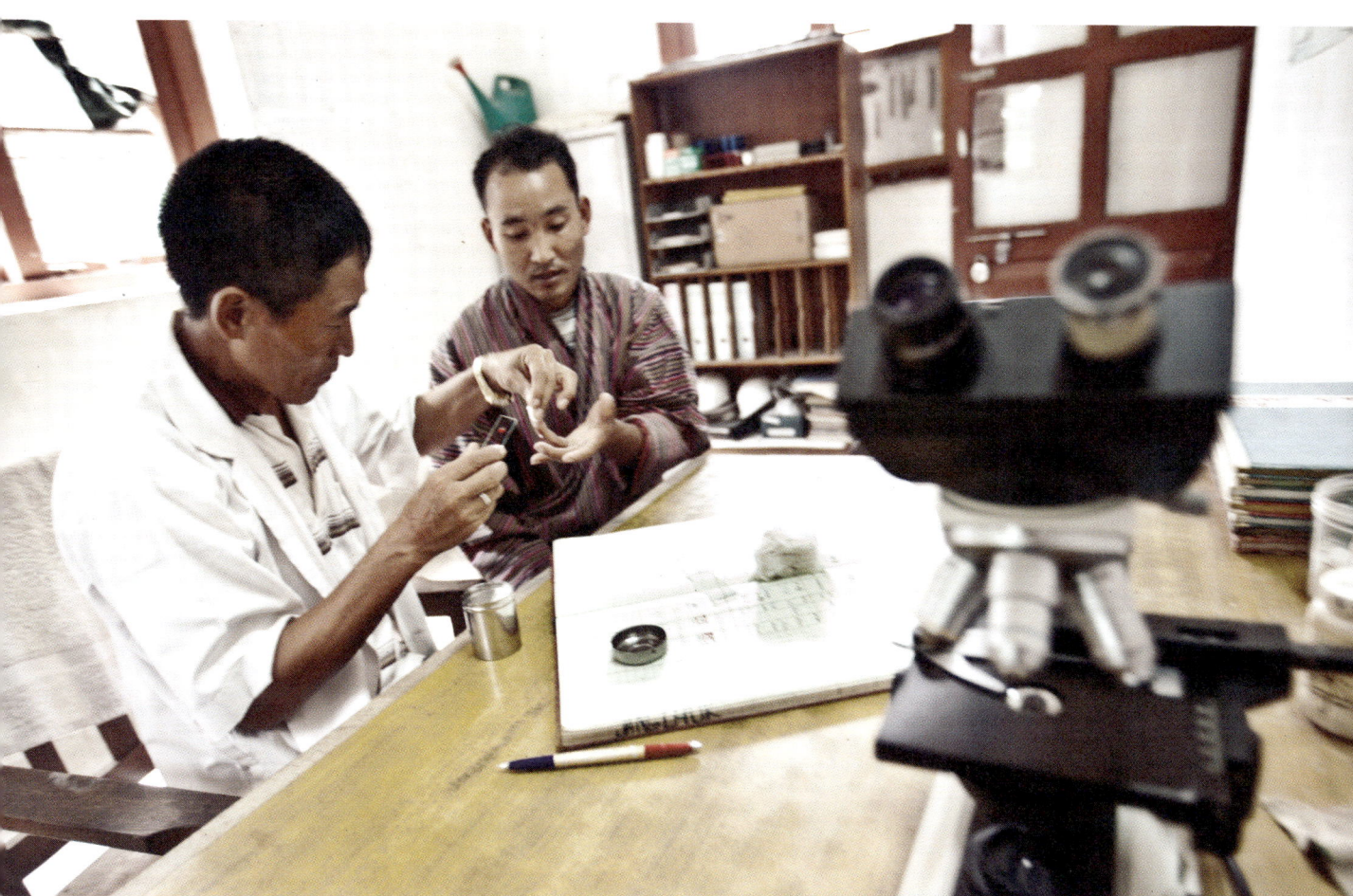

Box 2.3: Comparison of some important vectors outside of Africa

Region	Species	Resting location	Feeding time	Feeding location	Host preferences	Breeding sites
Europe and Middle East	An. sacharovi	Inside and outside	Peak 20:00–22:00	Inside and outside	Human and non-human	Typically large brackish marshes but also other habitats
	An. subpictus	Inside and outside		Inside and outside	Domestic animals and humans	Muddy pools often near houses. Also in barrow pits, buffalo wallows and artificial containers
South and South-East Asia	An. dirus	Mainly outside	Mainly late (20:00–02:00 hrs.)	Inside and outside	Mainly human	Small shady pools mainly in forests and plantations, footprints, stream seepages, wheelruts, gem pits, hollow logs, sometimes wells
	An. minimus	Mainly outside	All night	Inside and outside	Human and cows	Streams in forest foothills
	An. stephensi	Mainly inside	Late evening and night	Inside and outside	Mainly cattle and domestic animals	Urban vector: domestic water tanks and containers, construction sites Rural vector: clean water, river margins, rice fields, man-made pits and pools
	An. culicifacies	Mainly inside	Late evening and night	Inside and outside	Mainly cattle and domestic animals	Rural vector: clean water, river margins, rice fields, man-made pits and pools
	An. fluviatilis	Inside and outside	Peak 21:00–03:00 hrs.	Mainly inside	Human and non-human	Grassy edges of slow moving streams, springs, irrigation channels, sometimes in the edges of swamps and lakes

| GLOBAL OVERVIEW OF MALARIA EPIDEMIOLOGY |

Box 2.3 Comparison of some important vectors outside of Africa (continued)

Region	Species	Resting location	Feeding time	Feeding location	Host preferences	Breeding sites
Oceania	*An. farauti*	Mainly outside	Peak 20:00–21:00 and 23:00–03:00 hrs.	Mainly outside	Human and non-human	Emergent, floating and submerged vegetation in heavy shade. Also brackish pools, lagoons, and mangrove swamps in costal areas.
	An. punctulatus	Mainly outside	Peak around midnight	Mainly inside	Human and non-human	Sunny, temporary pools such as road ruts, footprints, margins of streams, and sloughs.
Central and South America	*An. albimanus*	Mainly outside, some inside	Late evening	Inside	Domestic animals (cattle, horses) 80%, humans 20%	Stagnant water, flooded pasture, or water with 25% emergent vegetation coverage
	An. darlingi	Inside and outside	Throughout the night but with biting peaks at dusk and dawn	Mainly Inside	Humans	Breeding sites and epidemics associated with deforestaiton and mining

Source: WHO 2005 (*19*), Sinka et al 2012 (*20*).

Map 2.3
Distribution of dominant or potentially important malaria vectors

A wide range of primary vectors exists globally. They are usually the target of most control efforts.

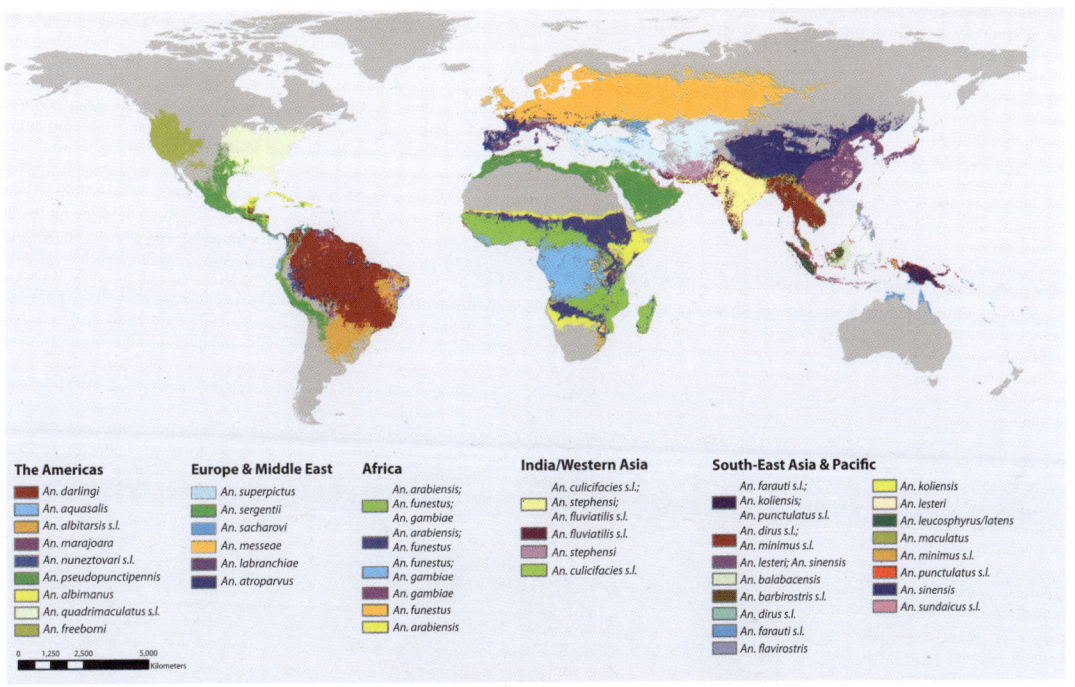

Source: Malaria Atlas Project (*17, 18*).
Map production: Public Health Information and Geographic Information Systems (GIS) World Health Organization.

The two most important methods of vector control are ITNs and IRS. ITNs are particularly effective against mosquitoes that bite late at night while people are sleeping under the treated net and IRS is effective against mosquitoes that bite and rest indoors. ITNs and IRS are much less effective against species that bite and rest outdoors such as the forest vector *An. Dirus*, which is widespread in Southern Asia. For these vectors, alternative strategies such as insecticide-treated hammocks and the use of personal repellents are sometimes employed. Some species with readily identified and accessible breeding sites, such as the urban vector in India *An. stephensii*, can be controlled using larvicidal technologies (spraying of larvicides or deploying fish which eat *Anopheles* larvae). Thus, vector control for settings outside of Africa must be carefully chosen to suit the circumstances prevalent in a country.

Because there is much variation in the behaviour of vectors that carry malaria, and because *P. falciparum* and *P. vivax* have different characteristics, the epidemiology of malaria is highly variable across the world. This report examines the epidemiology of malaria, and progress of malaria control, in four geographical regions outside of Africa. The four regions illustrate the diversity of situations in which malaria is encountered and the challenges for control but it is acknowledged that the epidemiology of malaria is still highly variable within these regions.

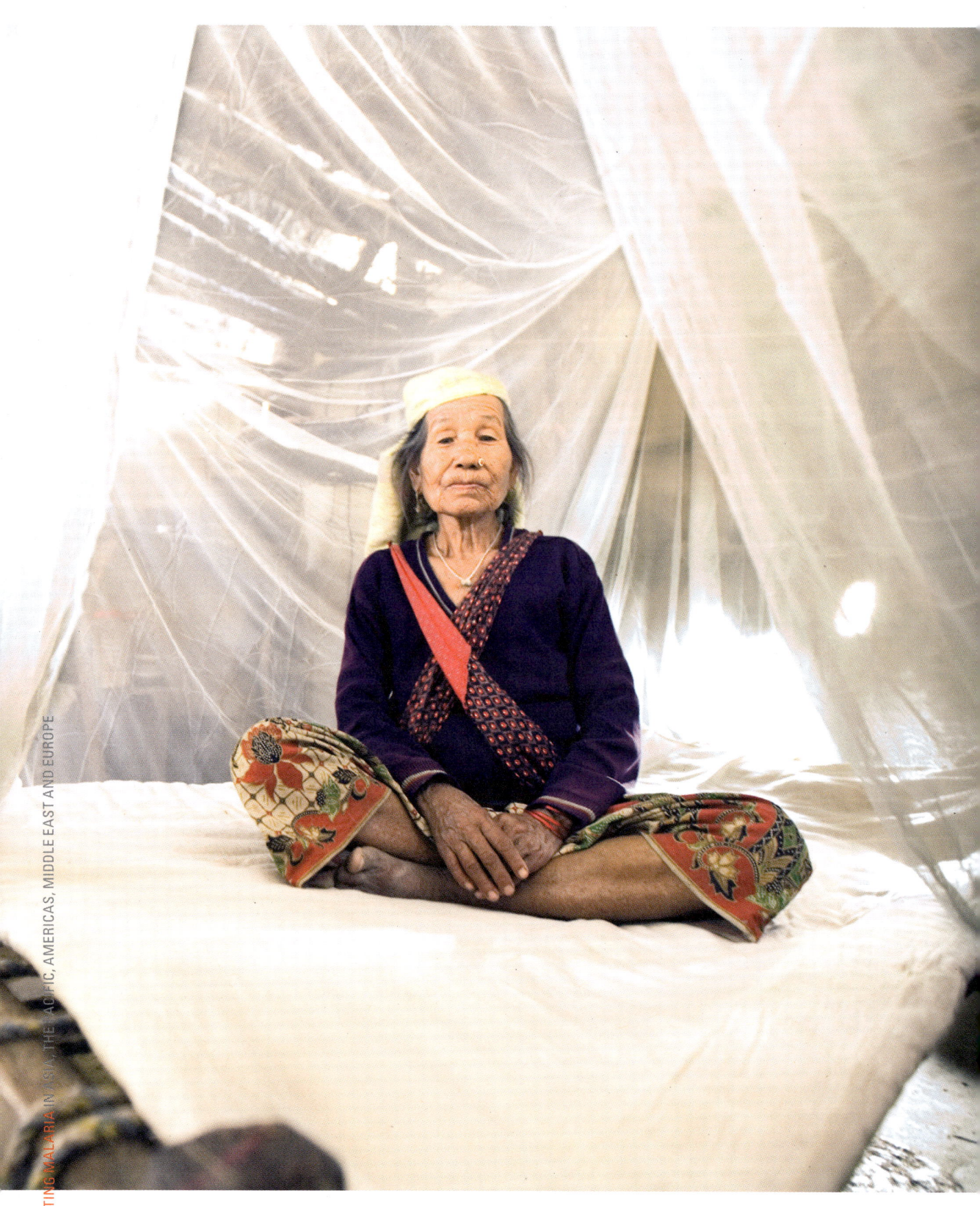

CHAPTER III

SOUTH AND SOUTH-EAST ASIA

Several countries in the region have been successful in reducing malaria, gains that are attributable to increasing the coverage of antimalaria interventions and to development activities which have made habitats less suitable for malaria vectors. But the region still contains the highest numbers of cases and deaths from malaria outside of Africa. Bringing down malaria in this region increasingly concentrates the disease in populations and areas that have been least affected by development—tribal populations and border areas—and where transmission can be particularly intense due to highly efficient vectors. Providing services to these areas and populations presents particular challenges and requires more commitment and resources than in easier-to-reach populations. Yet it is in these areas that efforts must be intensified in order to make significant inroads on the remaining burden of malaria and to prevent the emergence of drug resistance.

Countries in control phase: Bangladesh, Bhutan, Cambodia, China, India, Indonesia, Lao People's Democratic Republic, Myanmar, Nepal, Philippines, Thailand, Timor-Leste, Viet Nam

Countries in pre-elimination phase: Democratic People's Republic of Korea, Malaysia, Sri Lanka

Countries in elimination phase: Republic of Korea

Countries in prevention of reintroduction phase: None

Parasitological species of reported malaria cases: *P. falciparum* 58%, *P. vivax* 41%, *P. ovale*, *P. malariae*, and *P. knowlesi*

Main vectors: *An. Culicifacies* (in plains); *An. minimus*, *An. dirus*, *An. fluviatilis* (in forests); *An. stephensi* (in urban areas)

Population at risk: 2.1 billion; 62% of the resident population

Estimated number of cases: 29 million; 13% of global total, 84% of total outside of Africa

Estimated number of malaria deaths: 39 000; 6% of global total, 84% of total outside of Africa

Source: World Malaria Report 2011 (*16*).

| SOUTH AND SOUTH-EAST ASIA |

Epidemiological situation

Malaria transmission occurs in 17 countries of this region. Approximately 2 billion people in the region live at some risk of malaria, of which 525 million live at high risk (reported incidence more than 1 case per 1000 population per year). Most reported cases are due to P. falciparum although the proportion varies considerably by country; it exceeds 80% in the Lao People's Democratic Republic, Myanmar, Timor-Leste, and Viet Nam, while transmission is exclusively due to *P. vivax* in the Democratic People's Republic of Korea and the Republic of Korea (Map 3.1).

Map 3.1
Proportion of cases due to *P. falciparum* in South and South-East Asia, 2010

Malaria transmission occurs in 17 countries of this region. Approximately 2 billion people in the region live at some risk of malaria, of which 525 million live at high risk.

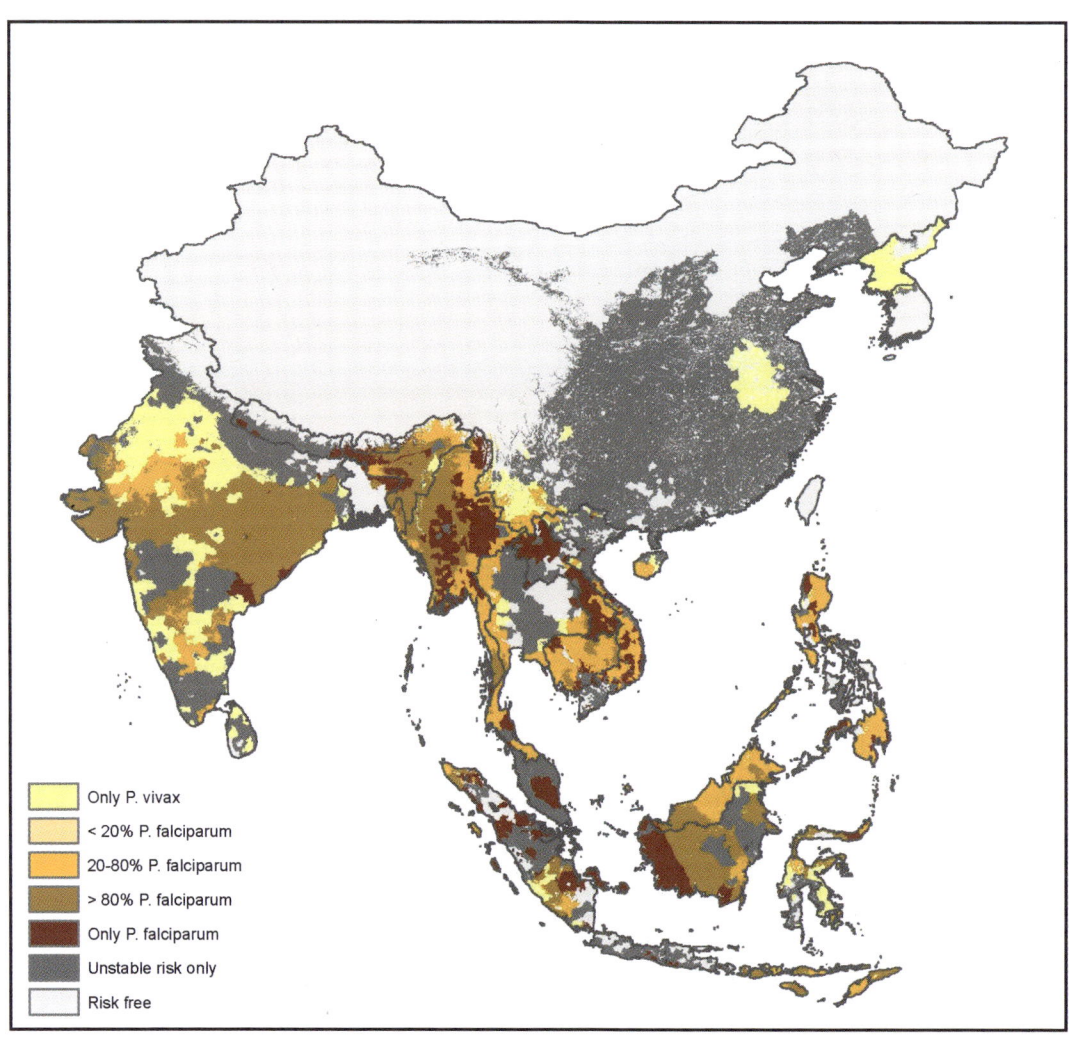

Note: Proportions are based on a four-year average of calculated annual parasite index for *P. falciparum* and *P. vivax* through 2010 and may not reflect the most recently reported subnational data.
Map production and source: Malaria Atlas Project (*17, 18*).

Development and population growth have led to rapid change over the past 50 years with urbanization and deforestation destroying many habitats suitable for malaria transmission. Control efforts have also increased, particularly in the last decade. During that time, decreases in the number of reported malaria cases have been seen in Bhutan, China, Democratic People's Republic of Korea, India, the Lao People's Democratic Republic, Malaysia, Philippines, Republic of Korea, Sri Lanka, Thailand, and Viet Nam (Figure 3.1). The Democratic People's Republic of Korea and Sri Lanka are now in the pre-elimination stage. There has been less progress in more populous countries with higher disease burdens, specifically Bangladesh, India, Indonesia, and Myanmar, although some progress has been documented subnationally with the Indonesian Islands of Java and Bali, which are aiming for elimination, as are several states of India. As malaria retreats it has become increasingly a problem of border areas, partly because these areas are less developed and have poorer access to health services but also because infections are introduced across borders (Map 3.2).

Figure 3.1
Trends in confirmed cases in South and South-East Asia

(a) Countries with more than 30 000 reported confirmed cases in 2010. India carries by far the heaviest burden of malaria among all countries in the region.

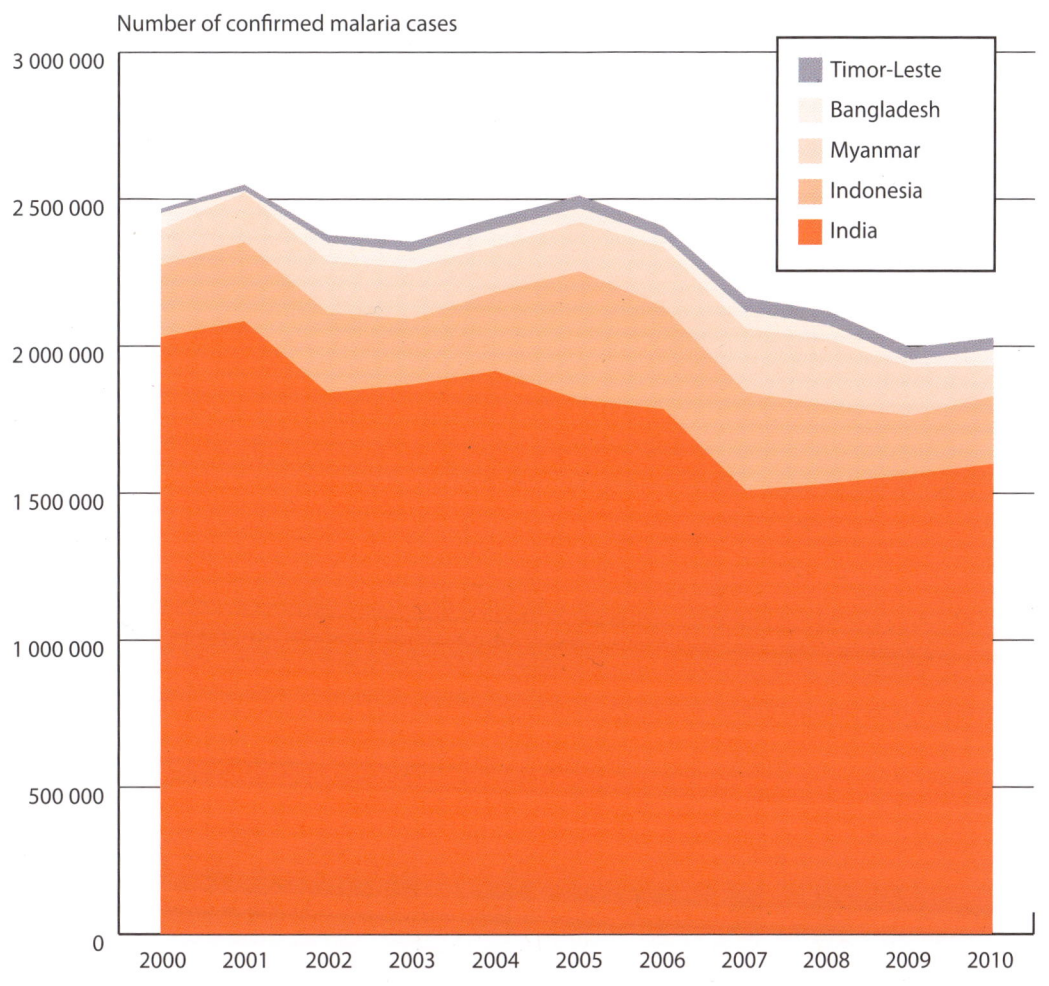

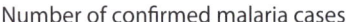| SOUTH AND SOUTH-EAST ASIA |

(b) Countries with less than 30 000 reported confirmed cases in 2010. Declines in confirmed cases from 2000 to 2010 were initially steep, particularly in Bhutan and the Democratic People's Republic of Korea, but by 2010 were more moderate.

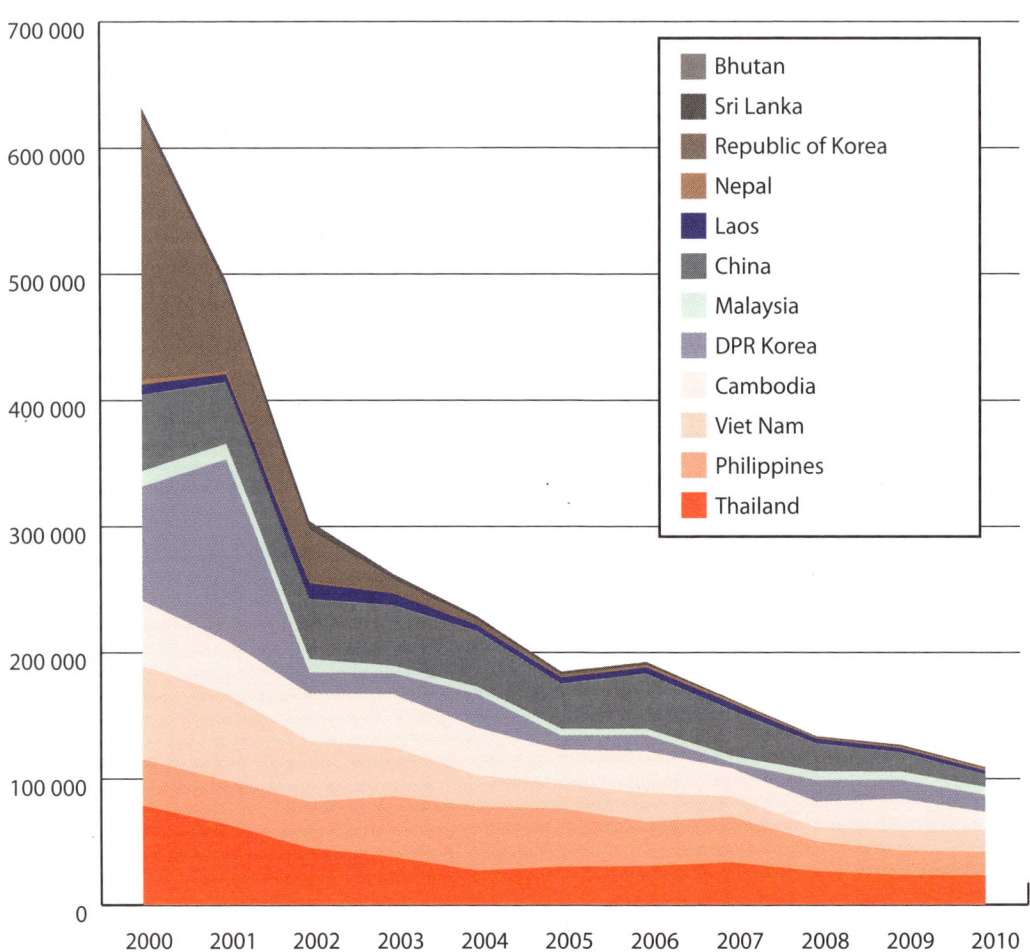

Source: World Malaria Report 2011 (*16*).

Map 3.2
Reported incidence of malaria by district in South and South-East Asia

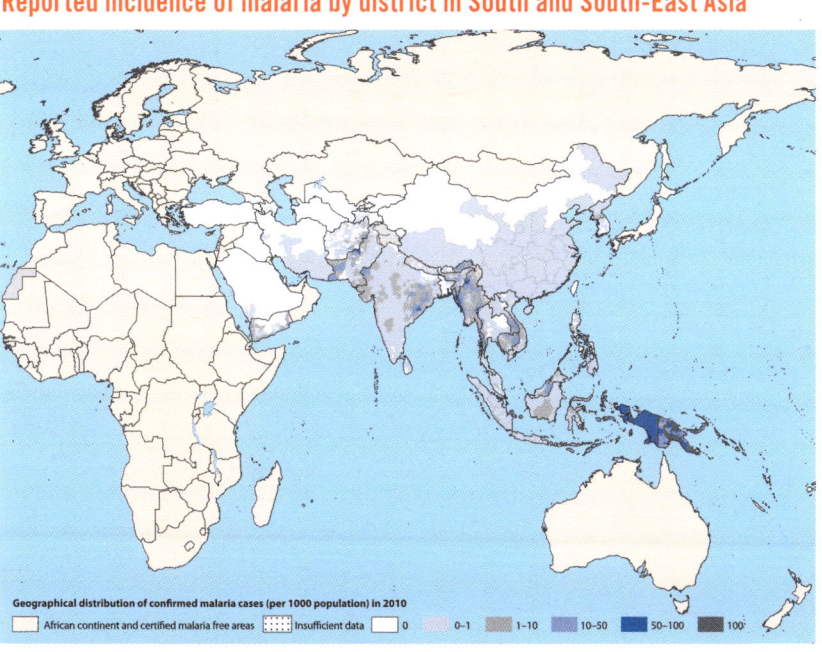

Data source: World Health Organization, 2010.
Map production: WHO Global Malaria Programme.

Populations affected

Malaria is principally found in the four following ecotypes:

- *Forest*. Malaria transmission in forested areas is intense due to the presence of highly efficient vectors. Indigenous tribal minorities represent a major risk group, often living in remote hilly areas with poor access to and utilization of health care facilities (the latter partly because of negative attitudes to modern medicine). Foothill areas provide good ground for cultivation of rice and other crops and are thus prone to deforestation and attract migrant workers who may have little immunity (*21*).

- *Plains*. These attract the largest concentration of human populations and are most intensely farmed. Malaria transmission is generally low and can be unstable leading to epidemics when climatic conditions are suitable.

- *Coast*. Coastal areas are also home to higher population densities. Malaria transmission can be intense in less developed areas because intervention coverage rates are often lower and opportunities are frequent for mosquitoes to thrive.

- *Urban*. Urban malaria is overwhelmingly confined to India, where it is associated with man-made structures containing water.

The different ecotypes have distinct epidemiologies even though they are sometimes separated by only short distances. For example, tribal populations living in forests in Orissa, India, have incidence rates that are almost 10 times higher than in the plains (Box 3.1). In forests, malaria is much more frequent in children under five years of age and declines with increasing age—an age pattern similar to that observed in Africa, in which adults have acquired immunity owing to frequent exposure during childhood. In the plains, malaria incidence rates do not decline

| SOUTH AND SOUTH-EAST ASIA |

with age, suggesting exposure to malaria was not sufficiently frequent to induce immunity. In Cambodia, populations living close to the forest are more likely to acquire malaria than those living at a distance (*22*). Malaria infection is associated with occupation and adult males have a higher risk of malaria infection than other population sub-groups, particularly where their activities lead them to stay overnight in forests for woodcutting, hunting, or gemstone mining. Poverty is a major driver for people to exploit forest resources where a high malaria risk exists.

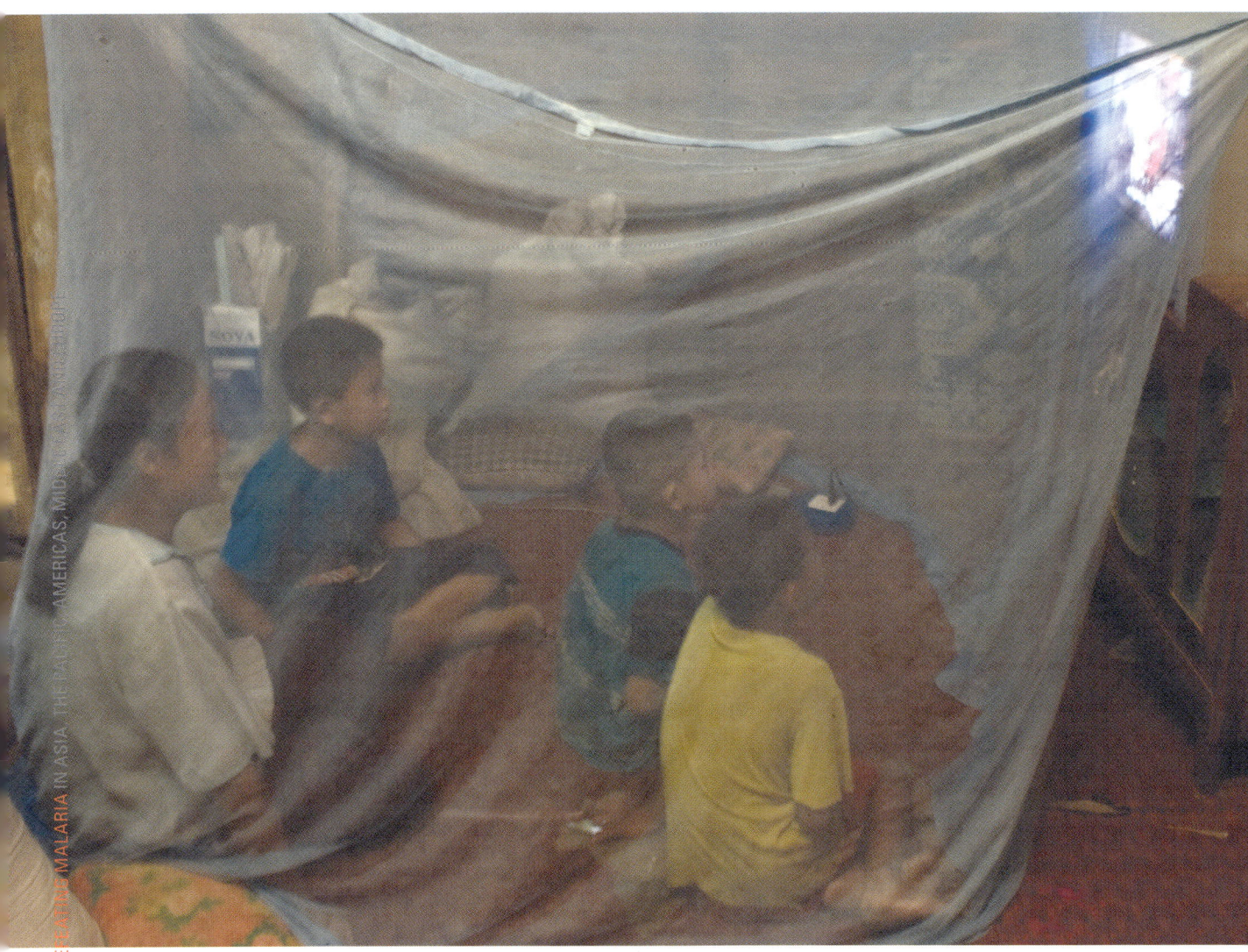

Box 3.1: Malaria in the plains and forests of Orissa, India

Orissa is one of the most highly malaria-endemic states in India, accounting for 24% of reported cases in 2010 despite consisting of less of than 4% of the national population. Malaria is particularly common among tribal groups which represent 44% of the population of Orissa. The incidence of malaria varies according to ecotype with forest areas having much higher incidence rates than plains areas (Figure 3.2). A study in Sundargarh District showed that forest areas had an annual incidence of 280 cases per 1000 population compared to 30 cases per 1000 on the plains (23). Approximately 84% of infections in forest areas were due to *P. falciparum* compared to 69% in plain areas. Such large differences occurred among villages in the two ecotypes that were separated by distances of only 10–15km.

A principal reason for the difference in malaria incidence by ecotype appears to be the vectors present. *Anopheles culicifacies* (sibling species C) is present in both ecotypes and is responsible for transmission year-round. It is not a very efficient vector, however, feeding mainly on animals other than humans; as a consequence, the number of infective bites delivered per year is small (0.009 and 0.014 infective bites per person per year in forest and plain areas respectively). In the forest areas an additional vector is present, *An. fluviatilis* (sibling species S), which feeds almost exclusively on humans. Even though it occurs with lower frequency than *An. culicifacies* it is responsible for 0.395 infective bites per person per year. In other words, 40% of the population are likely to be bitten by an infected *An. fluviatilis* in forest areas during a year, whereas less than 1% will be bitten by an infected *An. culicifacies*. In plains areas 1.4% of the population will be bitten by an infected *An. culicifacies* during a year while *An. fluviatilis* is not present.

The higher case incidence rates in forested areas are driven not only by more efficient vectors but also a larger reservoir of infection. Parasite prevalence surveys showed that 14% of the population in forested areas were infected with a malaria parasite (of which 76% were infected by *P. falciparum*) compared to 1.7% in plain areas (74% *P. falciparum*).

The different ecotypes are also associated with different age distributions of malaria. In forested areas malaria case incidence rates are highest in younger age groups and decrease in older ages. In the plains there is no correlation between malaria incidence and age. Forested areas thus exhibit case incidence rates and age distributions that are typical of sub-Saharan Africa in which older age groups acquire immunity after repeated malaria infections.

Tribal populations living in forested areas are poorer than those living in plain areas and have more limited access to preventive measures and health services. Since 2005, the National Rural Health Mission (NRHM) of the Government of India has been expanding health services to rural households all over the country, especially in the 18 least developed states of India. A key component has been to provide every village in the country with an accredited social health activist (ASHA) who is selected from the village itself. The ASHA collects blood samples for examination at clinics and provides treatment to positive cases. NRHM is also providing malaria treatment through mobile services in areas without access to clinics.

SOUTH AND SOUTH-EAST ASIA

Box 3.1. Malaria in the plains and forests of Orissa, India (continued)

Figure 3.2
The age distribution of malaria cases by forest areas and plains areas

Forested areas of India have many more malaria cases per person per year than do plains areas. In forested areas, those ages 1-4 years are particularly hard-hit.

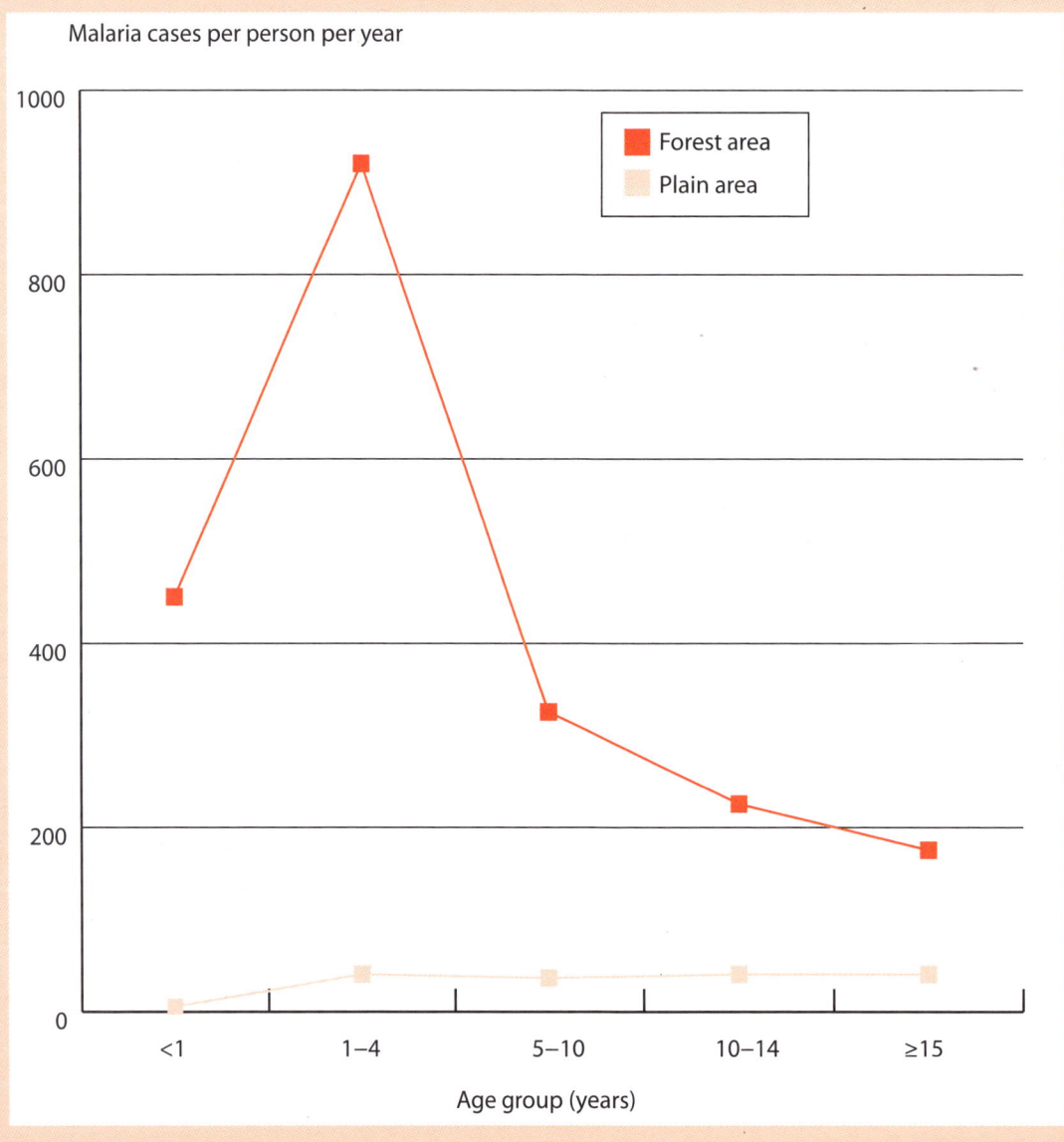

Source: Sharma SK et al 2006 (*23*).

Vectors: Vector behaviour contributes to the different epidemiologies observed. There are three highly efficient forest vector species in Asia, namely: *An. minimus*, *An. Dirus*, and *An. Fluviatilis* (*21*). *An. dirus* is a shade-loving deep-forest species: its archetypal breeding site is an elephant's footprint filled with dead leaves. It has a long lifespan and a strong preference for primate blood (and in forest villages, human are often the most abundant primates). Despite sometimes being responsible for less than 5% of bites it can still cause the majority of infections. *An. minimus* is associated with the forest-fringe and breeds in the pools formed at the edges of mountain streams which may have emergent or dangling vegetation. *An. minimus* is more common than *An. dirus* but has a shorter lifespan than and is more zoophilic. *An. fluviatilis* is associated with intense malaria transmission in forested areas of Orissa, India, and is commonly found around slow moving streams, springs, and irrigation channels. The species is mainly zoophilic and only moderately long lived. *An. culicifacies* is responsible for much of the transmission of malaria in plain areas but it is not an efficient vector. It is an endophilic mosquito with females feeding outdoors and often resting indoors. Because it rests on the walls of houses it is easily controlled by IRS. Larvae of *An. stephensi* are commonly found in man-made structures such as water tanks, roof gutters, and collections of water on building sites in urban areas.

Interventions: Development activities have had an important influence on malaria transmission over the years (*21*). In Kheda District, India, marshy land that sustained large populations of *An. culicifacies* was reclaimed for rice cultivation in the 1980s which led to a reduction in malaria transmission. In Indonesia, prawn and fish culture requiring high salinity proved injurious to *An. sundiacus*, thus eliminating its breeding in the coastal areas affected. Widespread deforestation in Asia has destroyed the habitats of some of the most efficient malaria vectors although in some cases natural forests may be replaced by oil palm plantations which are also associated with a high malaria risk (*24*).

Preventive measures have also contributed to malaria control. More than 150 million people in the region were protected with IRS in 2009; IRS covers more than 5% of the population at highest risk in Bhutan, Democratic People's Republic of Korea, India, Malaysia, Nepal, and Sri Lanka. Larvivorous fish are used in India, Indonesia, Myanmar, Sri Lanka, and Thailand. The number of ITNs distributed by national malaria control programmes between 2007 and 2009 was sufficient to protect approximately 70 million people with coverage potentially exceeding 10% in Cambodia, the Lao People's Democratic Republic, Malaysia, Sri Lanka, and Timor-Leste but in no case exceeding 20%. The apparent low coverage of preventive measures may be due to populations at risk being overestimated; when transmission is very focal the risk of transmission may be confined to only a small percentage of the population and preventive measures need to be targeted to ensure efficient use of resources (Box 3.2). It is also evident that populations acquire mosquito nets from sources other than national malaria control programmes and so are not accounted for in quantification exercises. These nets tend not to be treated with insecticide. Household surveys suggest that 80% of children under five years of age sleep under a mosquito net in Cambodia, the Lao People's Democratic Republic, and Viet Nam, but only a small percentage of these were treated with insecticide (ITNs) (*25*). Hence the national malaria control programmes have emphasized treating existing mosquito nets as well as distributing new ITNs in order to boost the proportion of the population that have access to them. This strategy differs from that practiced in most other regions of the world in which retreatment of nets has been discontinued owing to the introduction of long-lasting insecticidal nets (LLINs) which do not need retreatment.

| SOUTH AND SOUTH-EAST ASIA |

Box 3.2: Aiming to eliminate malaria in Bhutan

Bhutan has succeeded in driving down malaria in the past decade, with the number of reported confirmed cases falling from 5935 in 2000 to 436 in 2010. About 42% of Bhutan's 680 000 population is at risk of malaria. The populations at greatest risk are those that live in forest and forest-fringe settlements, especially where irrigation and development projects are present. In 2010, about 65% of cases were due to *P. vivax* 35% were due to *P. falciparum*.

Figure 3.3
Large decrease in the number of confirmed malaria cases reported in Bhutan, 2000–2010

Bhutan has made excellent progress since 2000 in reducing its malaria burden, having decreased the number of cases from 5935 that year to 436 in 2010.

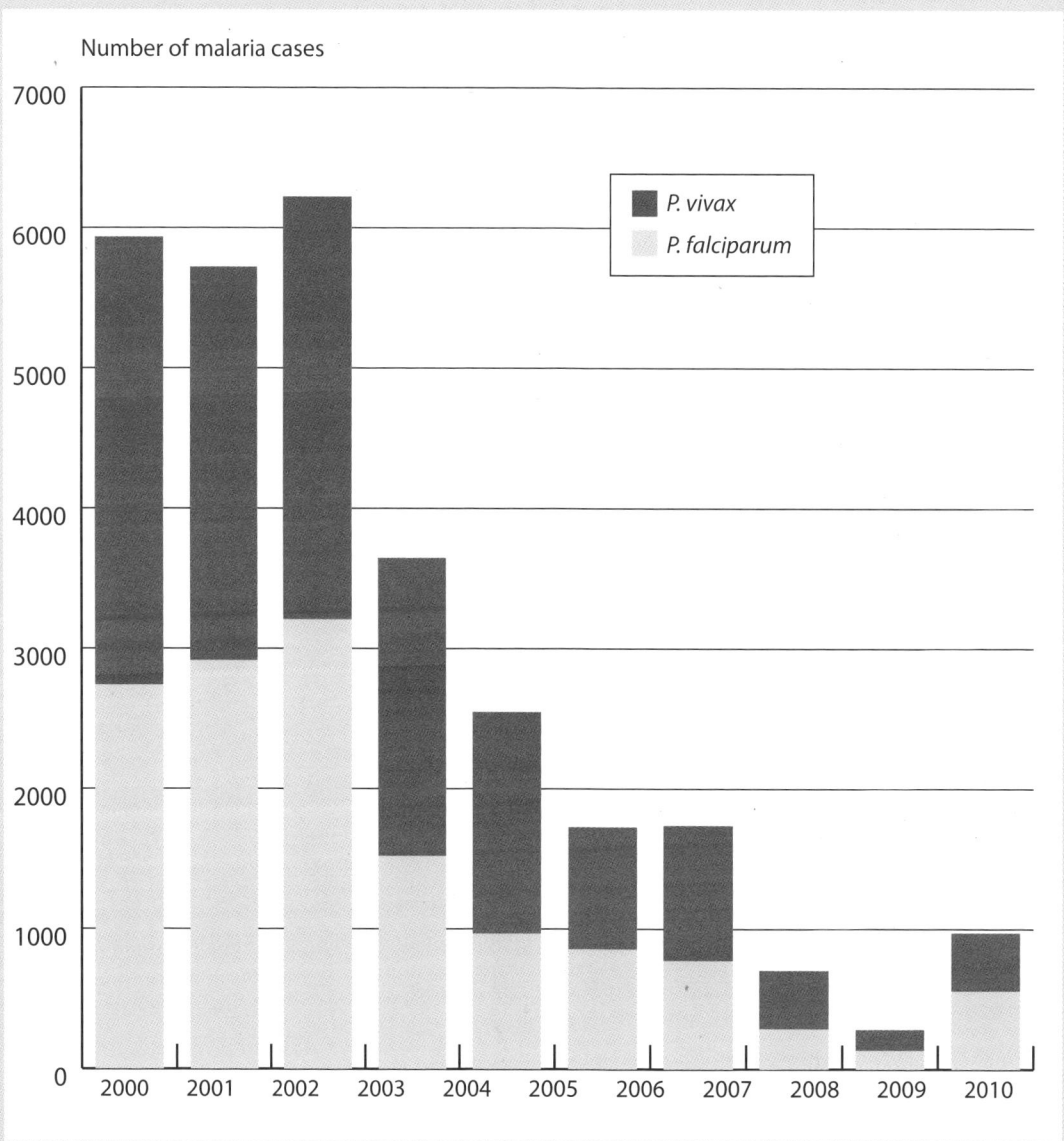

Source: Bhutan NMCP.

The Vector-borne Disease Control Programme (VDCP) of Bhutan coordinates and oversees the district health teams that execute all prevention activities related to vector-borne diseases. Bhutan's national health system feeds the VDCP critical information on the availability of commodities for malaria preventive activities and the number of cases detected and treated (26). The information guides malaria service delivery which is conducted by multipurpose malaria health workers known as "malaria technicians" (27) who work exclusively on malaria-related activities. They support vector control operations (IRS and LLIN distribution, entomological surveillance) and are responsible for undertaking diagnostic testing, providing malaria treatment, reporting malaria cases, and following up on case outcomes. The VDCP has recently begun to integrate malaria technicians into other vector-borne disease programmes, subsequently expanding these technicians' roles beyond malaria control. So far only a minority of technicians has begun this integration and the policy is being monitored to assess whether or not it will reduce the quality of malaria services delivered (28).

Indoor residual spraying (IRS) served as the country's main vector control method until 1998, when IRS activities halted and insecticide-treated nets (ITNs) became the primary vector control intervention. Starting in 2004, IRS was slowly re-introduced in areas that exceeded thresholds for malaria case incidence rates and occurrence of malaria deaths (28). In 2006, Bhutan began to distribute long-lasting insecticidal nets (LLINs) alongside targeted IRS.

The VDCP has addressed the needs of each malaria species in terms of diagnostic and treatment services. In 2006, the VDCP started using bivalent RDTs, which allow for the simultaneous testing of both *P. falciparum* and *P. vivax* with a single device (28). There are separate treatment protocols for *P. falciparum* and *P. vivax*. For *P. vivax* in adults, standard treatment consists of primaquine for 14 days followed by 3 days of split chloroquine doses. A 28-day clinical follow-up to measure medicine adherence and efficacy in each *P. vivax* case has been proposed. For *P. falciparum*, ACT was introduced as the first-line drug in 2006, and primaquine was recommended as a supplementary drug (as an anti-gametocyte) in 2011. All confirmed *P. falciparum* infections in Bhutan require a three-day compulsory hospital stay to ensure that patients receive directly observed therapy of their medications and daily blood slides. Upon discharge, patients are requested to return for a blood slide examination three days later and a malaria technician is dispatched to the patients' home if they fail to return.

Bhutan added malaria as a nationally notifiable disease in 2010. The country is also planning the implementation of active case detection (ACD), to be initiated in 2012. ACD activities will target high risk populations such as construction sites and seek to identify imported and asymptomatic infections and ensure diagnosis and treatment for all malaria-infected persons.

Several factors have contributed to Bhutan's great progress towards eliminating malaria. Health infrastructure is well developed and substantial funding for its health system is available through government financing and donor-backed development grants (29, 30). Hence, Bhutan has the resources to support an efficacious national surveillance system and extensive malaria case management activities. Bhutan also benefits from a sizeable and reliable health workforce (31), as well as a highly functional national supply and logistics system; in fact, no anti-malarial drug stock-outs have been recorded in Bhutan in recent years (26). Finally, Bhutan targets the distribution of LLINs and IRS to areas at highest risk of malaria, as an efficient use of commodities and resources. The approach is likely to be more sustainable for the long-term goal of malaria elimination than less targeted distribution of interventions.

| SOUTH AND SOUTH-EAST ASIA |

Box 3.2. Aiming to eliminate malaria in Bhutan (continued)

Bhutan has a national strategic goal to eliminate malaria by 2016 (*32*). While great progress has been made, several challenges remain. The eastern Himalayas present a challenging terrain with transportation made difficult in some seasons owing to landslides and road closures which result in reduced access to at-risk populations. Financing of the workforce and malaria activities must be maintained in order to ensure access to control measures. The country must also expand resources and capacity for monitoring antimalarial drug and insecticide resistance to ensure an arsenal of effective tools for treatment and prevention.

Lastly, and perhaps most importantly, significant numbers of cases are imported from the Indian states of Assam and West Bengal (*33*). With large numbers of migrant workers entering Bhutan to work on a growing number of large-scale development projects, the risk of continual re-introduction of malaria into these areas remains high. The number of imported infections is variable comprising 13% of the total confirmed cases in 2009 and 6.4% in 2010. The district of Sarpang, located alongside India's Assam state, has recorded the majority of Bhutan's imported cases over the last decade and trends in this district generally mirror trends in Assam. A comprehensive and practical cross-border malaria strategy with India would allow for communication and alignment of vector control operations in order to protect both sides of the border.

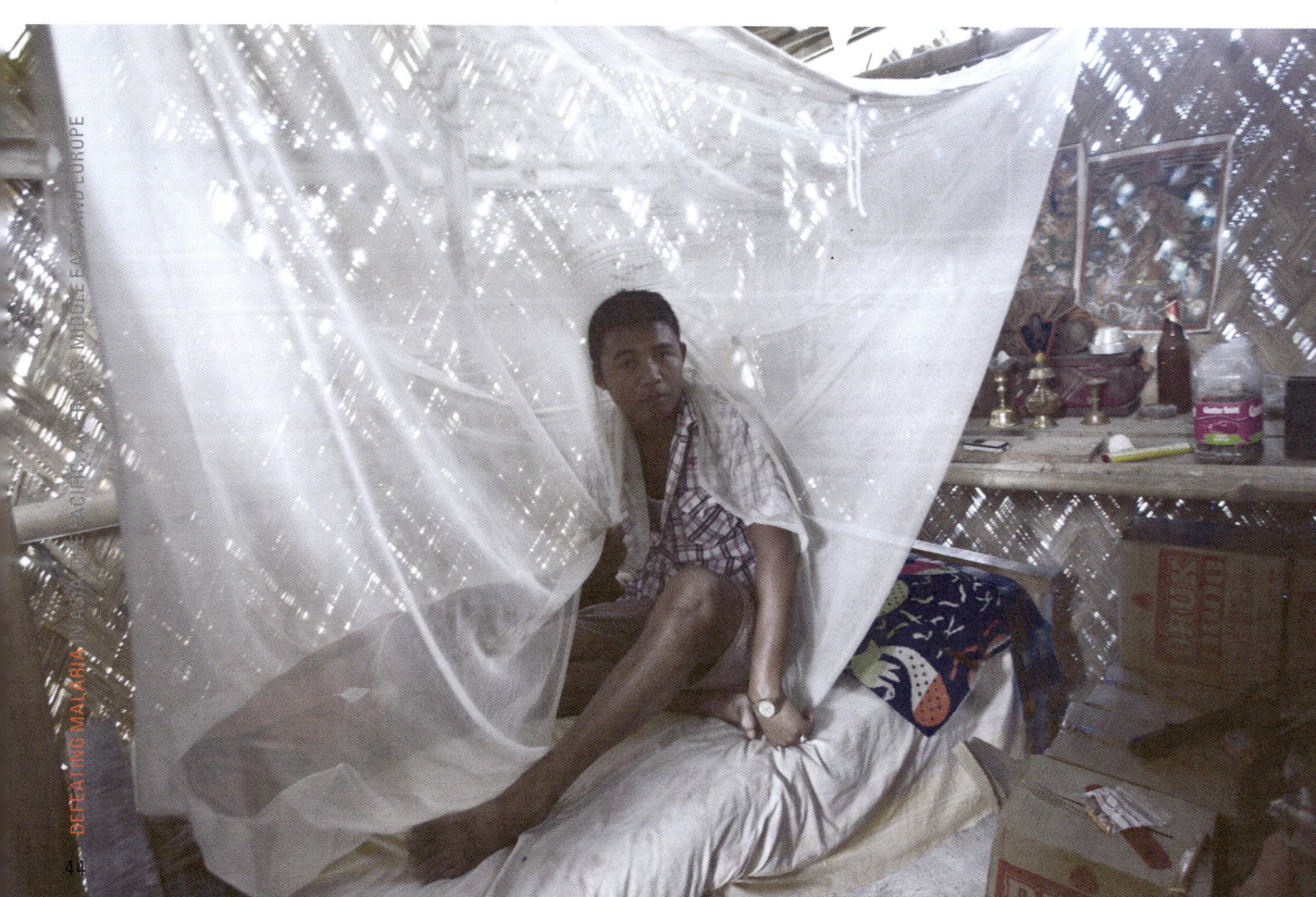

Public health services in the region generally aim to provide a parasite-based diagnosis using microscopy or RDTs and all countries with *falciparum* malaria have adopted ACTs. However, in Bangladesh, Cambodia, India, and Indonesia, more than half of fever cases are treated in the private sector, where the quality of diagnosis and treatment is variable. Since many of the populations most affected by malaria are located in areas not served by either public or private services, several countries have developed extensive programmes for community-based malaria diagnosis and treatment through volunteers in high-risk areas.

Counterfeit and substandard antimalarial medicines including artesunate are in circulation throughout the Mekong subregion and the problem is more pronounced in border areas. National governments and WHO are cooperating with Interpol to take action against organized criminals involved in counterfeiting. In addition, oral artemisinin-based monotherapies are also widely available, which are thought to contribute to the emergence and spread of resistance to artesunate that was reported in 2009 on the Cambodia-Thailand border. A multinational containment effort has started, involving tight regulation and education of private sector providers, education of the public, intensification of preventive measures, and close surveillance of potential cases of drug resistance. More recently, WHO, together with Roll Back Malaria, launched the *Global Plan for Artemisinin Resistance Containment* to address and provide guidance on this public health threat.

Resistance to the insecticides used to control mosquitoes is widespread, although vector control tools are currently effective in the vast majority of settings. In May 2012, WHO released the *Global Plan for Insecticide Resistance Management*, which outlines the pillars of action required to confront and overcome this threat, many of which are already being implemented (Box 3.3).

Summary

Several countries in the region have been successful in reducing malaria, partly due to increasing the coverage of antimalarial interventions but also because of development activities which have made habitats less suitable for malaria vectors. Despite some progress, the region still contains the highest numbers of cases and deaths from malaria outside of Africa. As malaria transmission has been controlled it is increasingly concentrated in populations and areas that have been least affected by development such as tribal populations and border areas, and where transmission can be particularly intense due to highly efficient vectors. Provision of services to these areas and populations presents particular challenges and requires more commitment and resources than in easier to reach populations. Yet it is in these areas that further efforts must be made in order to make significant inroads on the remaining burden of malaria outside of Africa and to prevent the emergence of drug resistance.

| SOUTH AND SOUTH-EAST ASIA |

Box 3.3: Resistance to antimalarial medicines and the insecticides used to control mosquitoes

Antimalarial medicines: Artemisinin-based combination therapies (ACTs) are critical to the future of malaria control programmes worldwide. ACTs are recommended by WHO as the first-line treatment for uncomplicated *falciparum* malaria, and the scale-up of these highly effective medicine combinations has been integral to the success of malaria control. No other antimalarial medicines are available at present with the same level of efficacy and tolerability as ACTs, and the earliest that such replacement medicines could be available is 2016.

P. falciparum resistance to artemisinins has been detected in Cambodia, Myanmar, Thailand, and Viet Nam. Of these countries, Myanmar has by far the greatest malaria burden with over 40 million people, or an estimated 69% of the Myanmar population, resident in malaria-endemic areas. Although the large majority of patients with delayed response to artemisinins are currently still being cured when treated with an ACT, resistance needs to be contained in existing "hotspots" before it is spread around the world, and the ability to treat *P. falciparum* malaria is lost worldwide. Such a scenario could result in a global resurgence of malaria-related illness and deaths, with major impacts on avoidable health spending, labour productivity, tourism, and economic growth. When resistance to previous generations of antimalarial medicines (e.g. chloroquine) emerged in the greater Mekong subregion and became widespread in the 1970s and 1980s, the number of malaria cases increased dramatically in many regions.

In January 2011, WHO released the *Global Plan for Artemisinin Resistance Containment*, which provided an urgent call to all stakeholders to maximize efforts to address this growing challenge to malaria control efforts worldwide.

Insecticides: Existing vector control tools are currently effective in the vast majority of settings. However, insecticide resistance has now been reported in nearly two thirds of countries with malaria transmission. It affects all major vector species and all classes of insecticides. Resistance to a class of chemicals known as pyrethroids seems to be the most widespread. Pyrethroids are the most commonly used chemicals for indoor residual spraying and are currently the only class available for use on long-lasting insecticidal nets. Resistance to the chemicals used in these tools could have a severe impact on the ability to maintain gains already achieved in reducing malaria or to aim for further success. In May 2012, WHO released the *Global Plan for Insecticide Resistance Management*, which outlined the pillars of action required to confront and overcome this threat, many of which are already being implemented.

Box 3.4: Asian Collaborative Training Network for Malaria

The Asian Collaborative Training Network for Malaria (ACTMalaria) is a collaborative training and information network with 11 country members: Bangladesh, Cambodia, China, Indonesia, the Lao People's Democratic Republic, Malaysia, Myanmar, Philippines, Thailand, Timor-Leste and Viet Nam. The network aims to provide training for member countries to meet the needs of malaria control in South-East Asia and the Mekong Delta and to improve communications between member countries. The network closely collaborates with technical partners and donors providing support to carry out the courses. ACTMalaria's vision is working together in sustained, equal partnership towards eliminating malaria as a major public health problem in the region.

Three major types of training are conducted by the network:

- Management of Malaria Field Operations, hosted by Thailand. This training aims to develop local capacity in malaria field operations.

- Broadening Involvement Team Training Workshop, hosted by Indonesia. This course aims to develop team members' ability to plan, implement, develop, and sustain a malaria control programme using evidence-based data gathered from scientific qualitative research, focus group discussions, and in-depth interviews.

- Transfer of Training Technology, hosted by Malaysia. This course aims to develop training teams that will improve the planning, implementation, development, and follow-up of national courses and international ACTMalaria courses.

Short training courses conducted by other countries include the anti-malarial drug policy and malaria surveillance and epidemic management training, conducted by China. Viet Nam hosted the pharmaceutical management for malaria training in collaboration with Management Sciences for Health and the insecticide resistance monitoring training in collaboration with the Institute of Tropical Medicine in Antwerp, Belgium. Cambodia hosted the training on in-vitro techniques to test *P. falciparum* and vector control management; the Philippines hosted trainings on operations research, training of trainers in judicious use of pesticides (in collaboration with the WHO Pesticide Evaluation Scheme), anti-malaria medicine quality monitoring (in collaboration with the US Pharmacopeial Convention), as well as instructional development skills and integrated vector management trainings.

The network aims to enhance relationships between member countries and partners through continuous sharing of knowledge and experience. The website (www.actmalaria.net) posts upcoming trainings and workshops offered by the network and other affiliated organizations. An electronic newsletter—ACTMalaria News—is published every two months and circulated to member countries and partners. The website also provides a portal for the ACTMalaria Information Resource Center which provides free online malaria resources to member countries, partners, and stakeholders of malaria in Asia and to every malaria-interested user. The center aims to be a one-stop source of online malaria information in Asia. This is a collaborative work of seven satellite libraries of some member countries that help build the collection through digitizing malaria resources.

ACTMalaria has contributed to the establishment of malaria microscopy quality assurance in the region. In collaboration with the WHO Western Pacific Region (WPRO), the WHO South-East Asia Regional Office, and the Australian Army Medical Research Institute, ACTMalaria has also served as a consultant on and conducted external competency assessment of malaria microscopy so countries can improve systems for quality assurance of malaria microscopy. ACTMalaria, the Research Institute for Tropical Medicine (RITM), and WPRO also initiated the establishment of the regional malaria slidebank based in RITM.

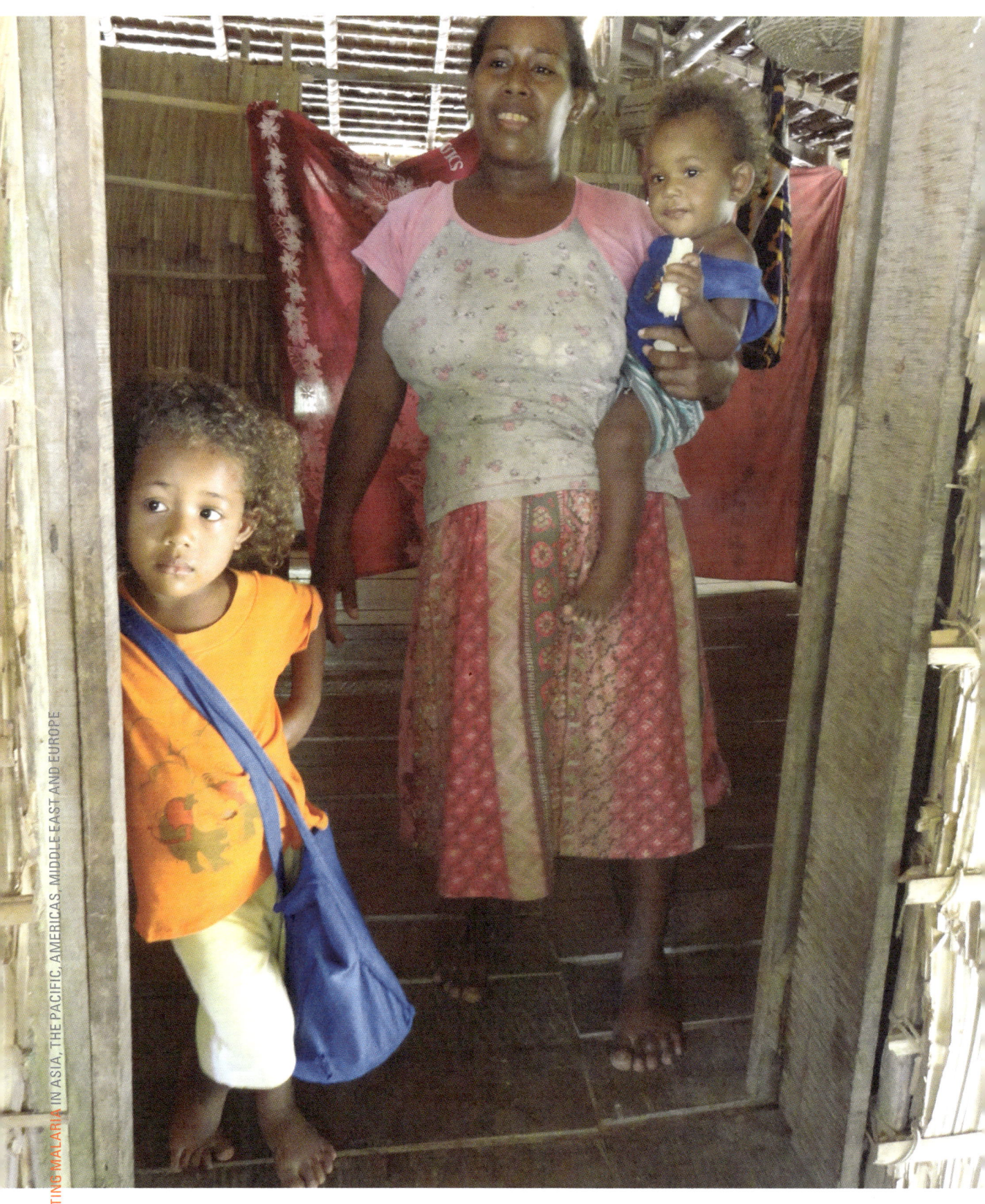

CHAPTER IV

OCEANIA

While some progress has been made in increasing access to malaria interventions, the disease remains a significant public health problem in much of the region. Some areas still have low coverage of preventive interventions and limited availability of parasitological diagnosis and appropriate medicines. The remoteness of many populations and health facilities presents additional challenges to combating the high levels of malaria transmission seen in the region. At the same time, the region is also rich in mineral and other natural resources which are increasingly being exploited to raise national government revenues. Ensuring that such revenues are invested in controlling a leading cause of morbidity and mortality is critical to securing prospects for further development.

Countries in control phase: Indonesia (Eastern Islands), Papua New Guinea, Solomon Islands, Vanuatu

Countries in pre-elimination phase: None

Countries in elimination phase: None

Countries in prevention of reintroduction phase: None

Parasitological species of reported malaria cases: *P. falciparum 63%, P. vivax 36%, P. ovale, P. malariae*

Main vectors: *Anopheles farauti* (coastal), *An. koliensis, An. punctulatus* (inland)

Population at risk: 7.6 million; 98% of the resident population

Estimated number of cases: 1.3 million; 0.6% of global total, 3.9% of total outside of Africa

Estimated number of malaria deaths: 3200; 0.5% of global total, 6.9% of total outside of Africa

Source: World Malaria Report 2011 (*16*).

| OCEANIA |

Map 4.1
Proportion of cases due to *P. falciparum* in Oceania, 2010

Malaria is a leading cause of morbidity and mortality in the eastern islands of Indonesia and the Pacific countries of Papua New Guinea, Solomon Islands, and, to a lesser extent, Vanuatu. The disease accounts for 10% of reported admissions to health facilities and 8% of deaths; most cases are due to P. falciparum.

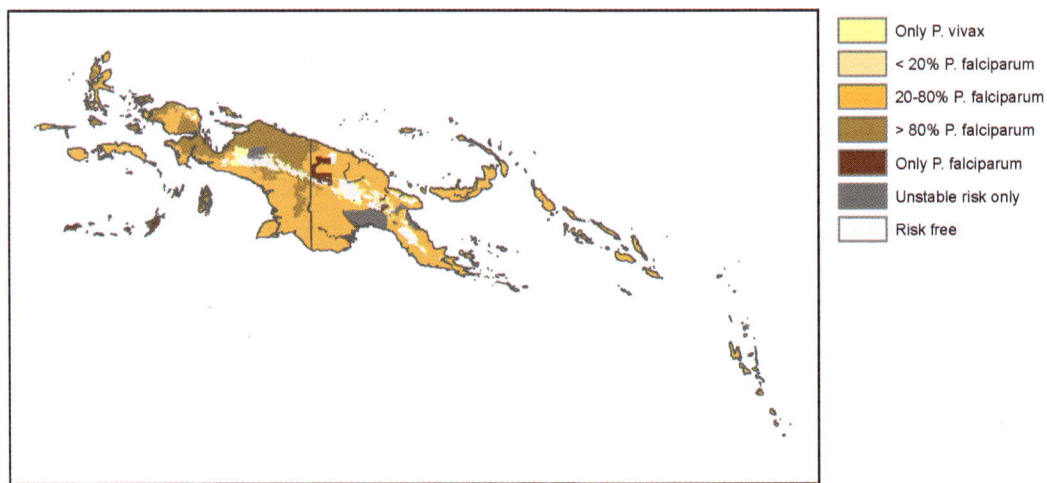

Note: Proportions are based on a four-year average of calculated annual parasite index for *P. falciparum* and *P. vivax* through 2010 and may not reflect the most recently reported subnational data.
Map production and source: Malaria Atlas Project (*17, 18*).

Epidemiological situation

Transmission is intense and widespread in the eastern islands of Indonesia and the Pacific countries of Papua New Guinea, Solomon Islands, and, to a lesser extent, Vanuatu.[f] Malaria is a leading cause of morbidity and mortality in these places accounting for 10% of reported admissions to health facilities and 8% of deaths. Most cases are due to *P. falciparum* but the proportion varies between countries (from 43% in Vanuatu to 79% in Papua New Guinea) and within countries with higher percentages of *P. vivax* found in the highlands of Papua New Guinea (Map 4.1) and eastern Indonesia.

Papua New Guinea has the largest population at risk and number of cases in the region but relatively few suspected cases receive a diagnostic test so reported confirmed cases appear fewer than in Indonesia. The two groups of islands, the Molucas and Papua of Indonesia, represent approximately 2% of the Indonesian population but account for almost 50% of reported cases in Indonesia. The number of confirmed cases has been relatively stable over the years apart from epidemic peaks. In the Solomon Islands intensive control measures helped to reduce cases and deaths during the 1990s but in 2000 civil unrest and interruption of health services led to a resurgence in the parts of the country affected. Cases have since decreased as services have been restored. Vanuatu has also seen a reduction in cases over the past decade. Efforts are being made to eliminate malaria from Temotu Island in the Solomon Islands and Tafeta in Vanuatu.

[f] Malaria does not occur in other Pacific islands owing to lack of mosquitoes capable of transmitting the malaria parasite.

Figure 4.1
Trends in confirmed cases in Papua New Guinea, Solomon Islands, and Vanuatu

Note that the increase in cases in Papua New Guinea in 2010, which affects the overall total, may be due to more patients receiving a diagnostic test rather than a real increase in the number of cases in the community.

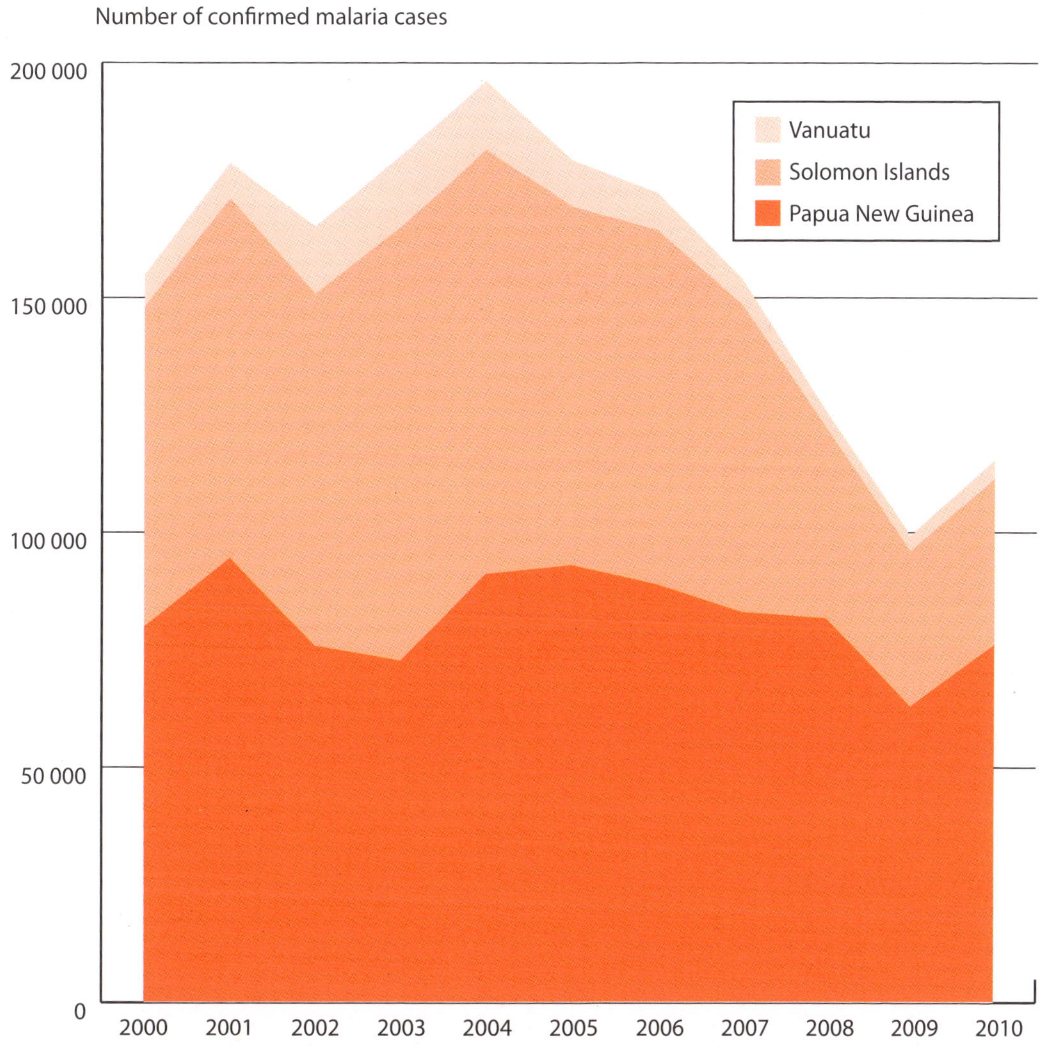

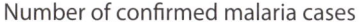

Note: Eastern islands of Indonesia not shown as subnational data is not available for all years from 2000 to 2010.
Source: World Malaria Report 2011 (*16*).

Populations affected

In coastal and lowland inland areas, malaria is highly endemic and the age and sex distribution of cases and deaths is similar to that of sub-Saharan Africa; the highest risk of illness and death is borne by children under five years of age and pregnant women, particularly those who are pregnant for the first time. In highlands areas, malaria transmission is less stable and populations have little immunity against malaria. The area is prone to epidemics associated with climatic events, such as those brought about by El Niño, with cases occurring in all age groups and a significant number of fatalities.

OCEANIA

Much of the region is characterized by low population densities and the remoteness of population groups which have traditionally been separated by mountain ranges, the sea, and other geographical barriers leading to great ethnic and linguistic diversity (there are more than 800 languages in Papua New Guinea alone which has a population of less than 7 million). Transport and communication remain difficult with little road infrastructure. Many inland villages are only accessible by air while coastal villages can be rendered inaccessible by rough seas at certain times of the year. The remoteness not only interrupts service provision but adds to the costs of delivering services. As transport and communications have improved, more people are exposed to malaria; people from highlands areas are exposed when visiting the coast and malaria has established itself in some low lying parts of highland areas. Climate warming is also considered to be a threat with the possibility of malaria becoming increasingly endemic in the lower areas of highlands regions.

Vectors
Two species of anopheline mosquito are responsible for most malaria transmission, namely *An. punctulatus* and *An. farauti* (*34*). Both are long living and highly efficient. *An. faurauti* tends to be found in low lying parts of valleys while *An. punctulatus* inhabits the slopes. *An. punctulatus* only breeds in fresh water sites which are exposed to the sun. *An. farauti* is tolerant to salt so can also breed in coastal areas. *An. farauti* is believed to have two biting peaks, one from 8–9 pm and another between 11 pm and 3 am. It has been observed that the second biting peak can be eliminated by spraying DDT (dichlorodiphenyltrichloroethane) so that the species only bites in the early evening, potentially rendering ITNs less effective.

Interventions
IRS is used extensively in Solomon Islands protecting approximately 45% of the population in 2010. IRS was used on a relatively small scale in Indonesia and Vanuatu in 2010 with 60 000 and 16 000 people protected respectively, and only for control of epidemics in the highlands of Papua New Guinea. ITNs are used widely, with the number of ITNs procured between 2008 and 2010 being sufficient to protect 35% of the population at risk in Papua New Guinea to 100% in Solomon Islands and Vanuatu.

ACTs have been adopted as the recommended first-line treatment for *P. falciparum* malaria in all countries but treatment practices in health facilities do not always follow policies. Also, the availability of diagnostic and treatment services is variable. In Solomon Islands and Vanuatu approximately 87% and 100% of reported suspected cases are tested and sufficient quantities of ACTs are procured to treat all patients attending public sector health facilities. In Papua New Guinea, less than 16% of suspected cases attending health centres and hospitals are tested and the quantities of ACTs procured are not sufficient to treat all cases attending health facilities. In eastern Indonesia, 62% of suspected malaria cases attending public health facilities receive a diagnostic test.

Summary
Despite some progress in the delivery of interventions, malaria remains a significant public health problem in much of the region. Some areas still have low coverage of preventive interventions and limited availability of parasitological diagnosis and appropriate medicines. The remoteness of many populations and health facilities presents additional challenges to combating the high levels of malaria transmission seen in the region. However, the region is also rich in mineral and other natural resources which are increasingly being exploited to raise revenues for national governments. It will be important to ensure that such revenues are invested in controlling a leading cause of morbidity and mortality so that further development can ensue.

Box 4.1: Endemic and epidemic malaria in Papua New Guinea

Malaria is a major public health problem in Papua New Guinea, accounting for approximately 11% of all health facility admissions and 8% of reported deaths. All four human malaria species are present. *P. falciparum* accounts for 81% of cases in coastal and island regions and 61% of cases in the highlands region; *P. vivax* is the next most common species with 17% in coastal and islands regions and 34% of cases in the highlands; while *P. malariae* accounts for 2% to 5% of cases. *P. ovale* is rare.

Malaria is highly endemic and comparatively stable in coastal areas where two-thirds of the population live. People in these areas are continuously exposed to malaria and have developed partial immunity protecting them from serious illness and death due to malaria. Cases and deaths are concentrated in younger age groups which have yet to develop immunity (Figure 4.2). Delivery of insecticide-treated nets (ITNs) to all households constitutes the main strategy for preventing malaria in these coastal and island areas.

Malaria is less stable in the Highlands Region, which is prone to epidemics with a significant number of fatalities. In the early twentieth century, there was practically no malaria in these areas. However, malaria cases are reported now in all parts of the highlands with a large proportion derived from people who have visited the coast. Because people in the highlands are infrequently exposed to malaria they do not get the opportunity to develop immunity. When they do contract malaria, the disease takes a virulent course, which may end in death. The age distribution of cases in the highlands largely reflects the degree of exposure. Because of intermittent transmission, special emphasis is placed on effective case management, particularly for severe malaria, as well as prophylactic drug administration to pregnant women and travelers to coastal areas. Indoor residual spraying is undertaken in areas below 1600 meters and there is increasing use of ITNs in areas capable of sustaining local transmission. Control of vector breeding through larviciding has its place in limited localities, such as industrial sites, urban centres, and new settlements.

| OCEANIA |

Box 4.1 Endemic and epidemic malaria in Papua New Guinea (continued)

Figure 4.2
Age distribution of severe malaria in the coastal, islands, and highlands areas of Papua New Guinea

In coastal and island areas malaria admission rates decrease with age partly because of the immunity developed as a result of continual exposure to malaria, although the trend is also affected partly by lower health service utilization rates in older age groups. Malaria admission rates in the highlands are highest in ages 15-44 partly because infrequent exposure in the highlands produces little immunity and persons in these age groups are more likely to travel to the coast where they acquire infection.

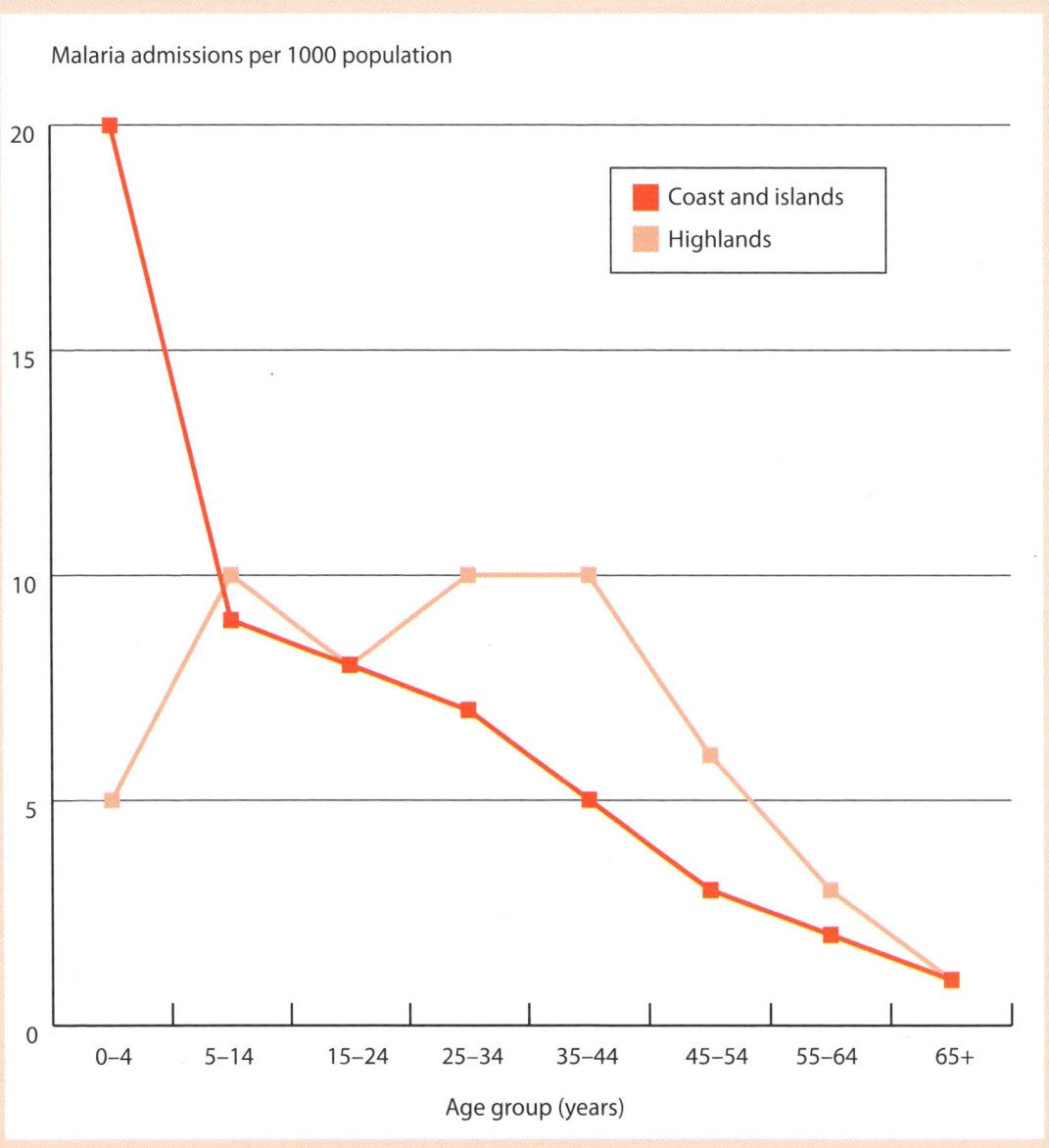

Source: Department of Health, Papua New Guinea.

Box 4.2: Asia Pacific Malaria Elimination Network

The Asia Pacific Malaria Elimination Network (APMEN) was established in 2009. It is a regional collaboration that supports countries in the Asia Pacific region that aspire to eliminate malaria. It comprises twelve countries: Bhutan, Cambodia, China, the Democratic People's Republic of Korea, Indonesia, Malaysia, the Philippines, the Republic of Korea, Solomon Islands, Sri Lanka, Thailand, and Vanuatu.

The countries share their experiences with new approaches and challenges in eliminating malaria and determine optimal ways to translate research and best practice into action. Programme managers work with a broad range of partners, including academic, development, nongovernmental, and private sector representatives to address the region's malaria challenges. The network features two working groups, the Vivax Working Group and the Vector Control Working Group. The Vivax Working Group catalyzes operational research and provides technical guidance on research projects. Both working groups identify gaps in skills and negotiate with partner organizations and agencies to tailor training and workshops to the needs of country partners with a specific focus on elimination. APMEN is supported by a Joint-Secretariat between the Global Health Group at the University of California, San Francisco, USA, and the School of Population Health, University of Queensland, Australia. APMEN currently receives foundation funding from the Australian Agency for International Development (AusAID).

The network features the following five focus areas with examples of this work:

- *Evidence generation.* APMEN's research grant programme provides funding for small to medium operational research projects by APMEN country researchers, with an emphasis on improved diagnostic and treatment tools for *P. vivax*.

- *Programme documentation.* APMEN works with country programmes to document and disseminate their experiences in eliminating malaria through case studies.

- *Capacity building.* APMEN fellowships provide funding for its country health professionals to pursue field work, professional development, and advanced training in other APMEN country institutions. In addition, APMEN has undertaken training for country partners on subjects such as geographic information systems, molecular genotyping, and the relevance and importance of glucose-6-phosphate dehydrogenase deficiency in the Asia Pacific region.

- *Information exchange.* Annual APMEN meetings bring together country partners to share challenges, best practices, and lessons learned. APMEN's topic-based working groups enable partners to delve deeper into technical issues and guide the network's malaria elimination agenda.

- *Advocacy.* APMEN advocates on behalf of the malaria-eliminating countries in the Asia Pacific region, taking on critical issues such as *P. vivax*, long-term financing for elimination, and cross-border importation of malaria cases.

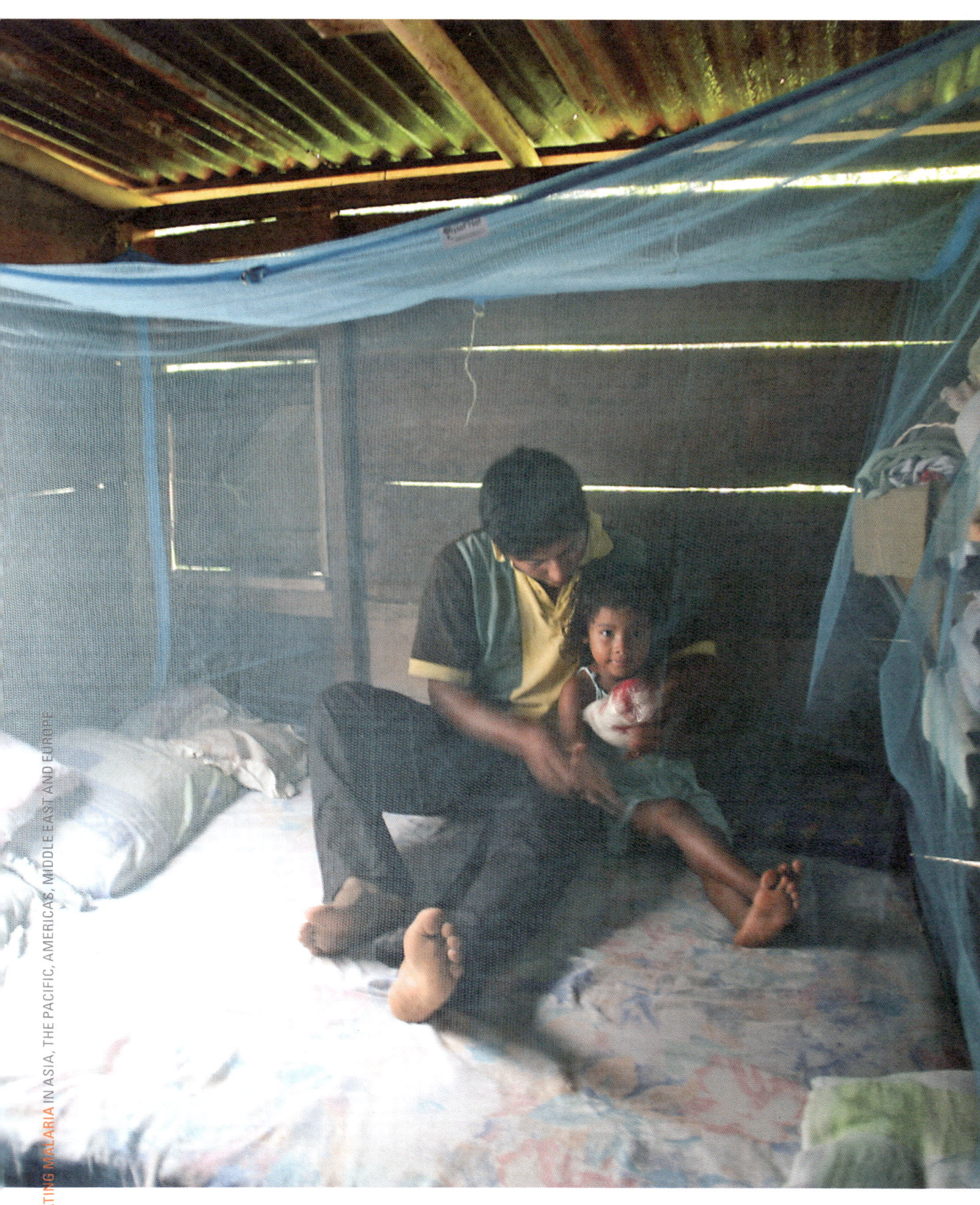

CHAPTER V

THE AMERICAS

Overall reductions in malaria cases and deaths in the Americas have resulted in considerable diversity in the status of control programmes within the region. Countries today span the spectrum of phases, including control, pre-elimination, prevention of reintroduction, and control in complex emergencies. Despite much progress, significant challenges persist among populations with the highest incidence: they have limited access to services, limited infrastructure, extreme poverty, and settlements in hard to reach, scattered, rural areas or marginal urban areas. Developing and implementing programmes that take into account these populations requires robust and durable political commitment and appropriate levels of finance.

Countries in control phase: Belize, Bolivia (Plurinational State of), Brazil, Colombia, Costa Rica, the Dominican Republic, Ecuador, French Guiana (France), Guatemala, Guyana, Haiti, Honduras, Nicaragua, Panama, Peru, Suriname, Venezuela (Bolivarian Republic of)

Countries in pre-elimination phase: Argentina, El Salvador, Mexico, Paraguay

Countries in elimination phase: None

Countries in prevention of reintroduction phase: Bahamas, Jamaica

Parasitological species of reported malaria cases: *P. falciparum 21%, P. vivax 79%, P. ovale, P. malariae*

Main vectors: *An. albimanus, An. darlingi*

Population at risk: 160 million; 29% of the resident population

Estimated number of cases: 1.1 million; 0.5% of global total, 3.3% of total outside of Africa

Estimated number of malaria deaths: 1200; 0.2% of global total, 2.5% of total outside of Africa

Source: World Malaria Report 2011 (*16*).

| THE AMERICAS |

Epidemiological situation

Malaria transmission occurs in 21 countries of the region with almost 3 out of every 10 persons at varying degrees of risk of malaria transmission. The number of confirmed cases reported in the region decreased by more than 40% from 1.18 million in 2000 to 669 000 in 2010 (Figure 5.1). In addition, 133 malaria deaths were reported in 2008, a decrease of more than 60% compared to 2000. Four countries—Argentina, El Salvador, Mexico, and Paraguay—are moving to eliminate malaria from within their borders. Malaria control programmes are in the process of reorientation to investigate every case of malaria and determine if it was acquired locally. Whereas most countries showed downward trends in malaria cases, three countries reported increases in the number of cases between 2000 and 2010 (the Dominican Republic, Haiti, and Venezuela) while the Bahamas and Jamaica, which had eliminated local transmission of the disease, experienced malaria outbreaks in the past decade.

More than three quarters of infections are caused by *P. vivax* and the percentage of cases due to *P. falciparum* is almost 100% in Haiti and the Dominican Republic.

Map 5.1
Proportion of cases due to *P. falciparum* in the Americas, 2010

Malaria transmission occurs in 21 countries of the region with almost 3 of every 10 persons at varying degrees of risk. More than three quarters of infections are caused by P. vivax *and the percentage of cases due to* P. falciparum *is almost 100% in Haiti and the Dominican Republic.*

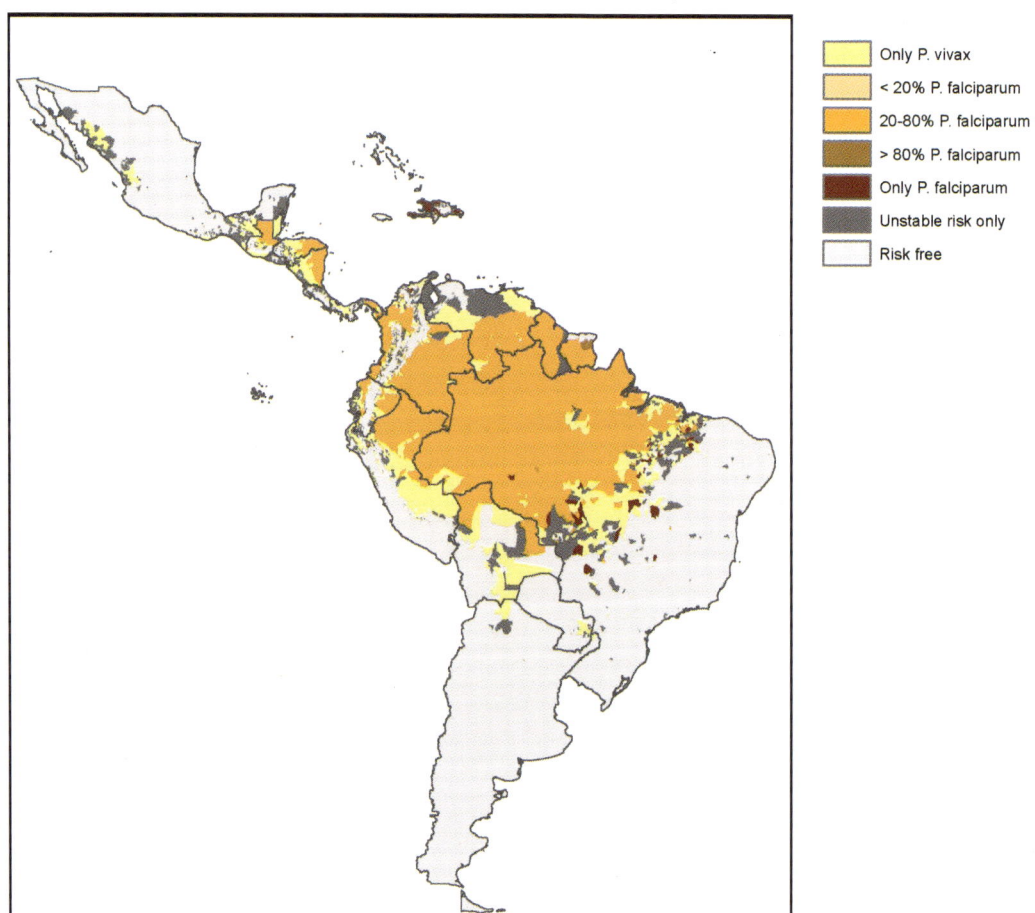

Note: Proportions are based on a four-year average of calculated annual parasite index for *P. falciparum* and *P. vivax* through 2010 and may not reflect the most recently reported subnational data.
Map production and source: Malaria Atlas Project (*17, 18*).

Figure 5.1
Trends in confirmed cases in the Americas

(a) Countries with more than 30 000 reported confirmed cases in 2010. Note that the increase in cases in Haiti in 2010, may be due to a combination of more people receiving a diagnostic test as part of earthquake relief efforts as well as weakened infrastructure resulting in favorable conditions for mosquito breeding.

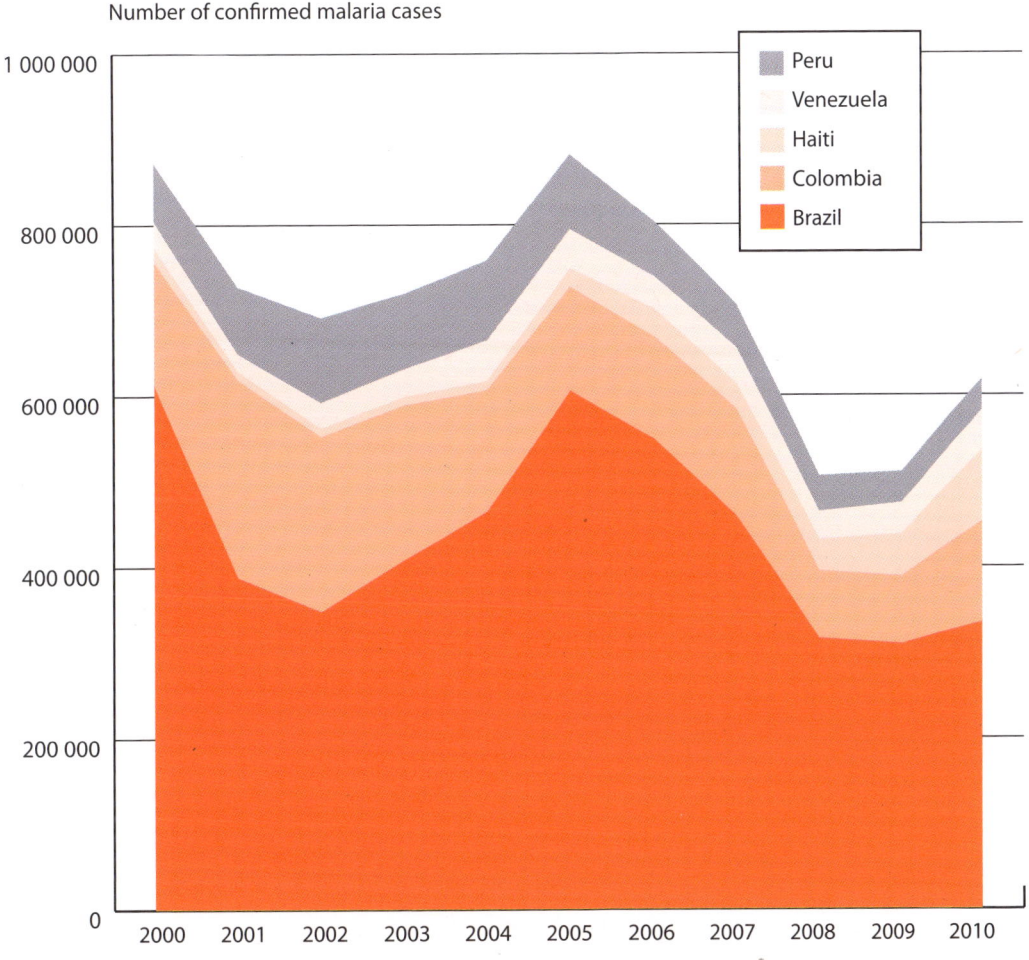

| THE AMERICAS |

(b) Countries with less than 30 000 reported confirmed cases in 2010. Many countries achieved steep declines early on in the last decade; these gains have been largely sustained since then.

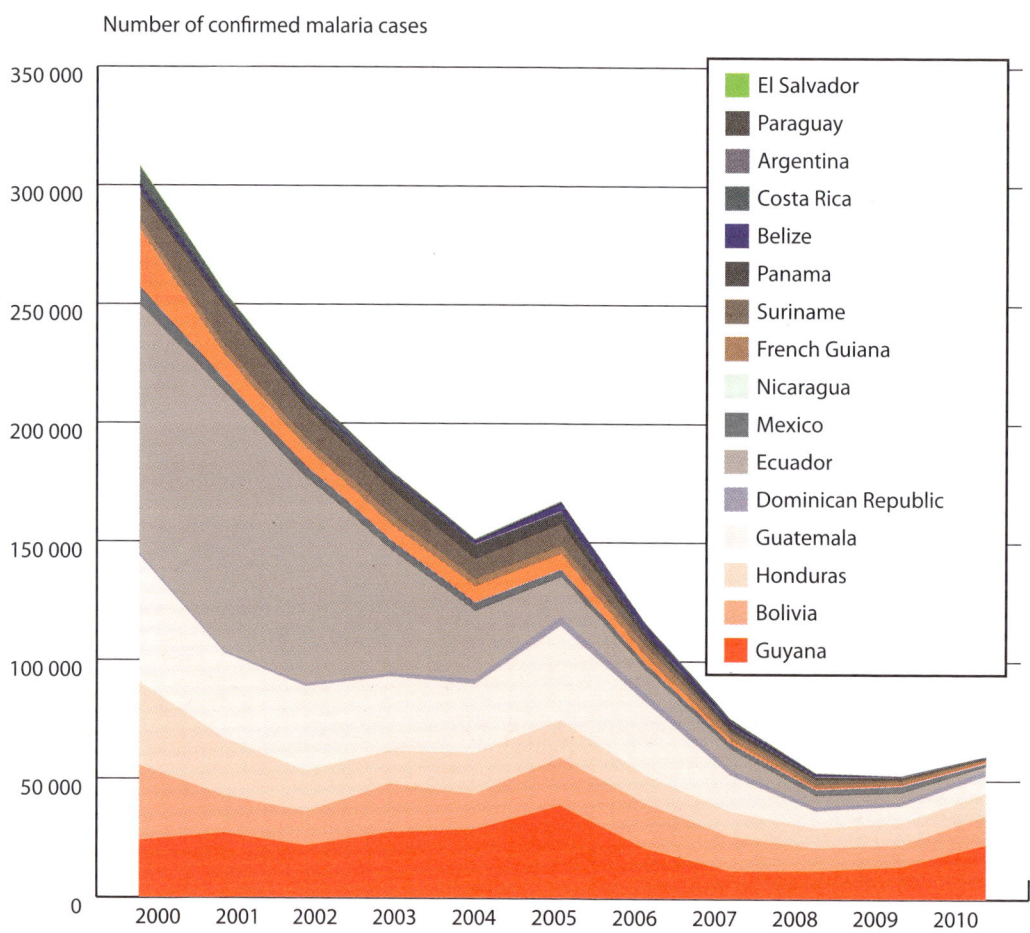

Source: World Malaria Report 2011 (*16*).

Populations affected

The majority of malaria cases arise from the Amazon Basin in districts of Brazil, Bolivia, Colombia, Peru, and Venezuela, where reported incidence rates frequently exceed 50 cases per 1000 population per year (*35*). Many infections are associated with settlement projects, mining activities, and forestry and a collaborative effort to tackle the disease is under way (Box 5.2).

In Anajas Municipality in Brazil, which has the highest recorded incidence rate in the region (452 cases per 1000 inhabitants per year), transmission is associated with palm harvesting. In the departments of Beni and Pando in the northern part of Bolivia, the highest concentration of cases in the country is found in areas of chestnut harvesting, while in Guyana and eastern Venezuela cases are associated with gold mining.

Box 5.1: Malaria control in Suriname

The ecological environment of Suriname is largely Amazonian rain forest. Approximately 65 000 people are estimated to be at risk. Malaria is mainly a problem inland where Amerindians and Maroons live in tribal communities, and where migrant workers are active in small-scale gold mining. Most of these migrant workers lack entry permits, creating other unique malaria control challenges.

Figure 5.2
Distribution of *P. falciparum*/mixed and *P. vivax*/*P. malariae* cases in Suriname, 2004–2010

As cases of malaria in Suriname have been reduced, the proportion due to P. vivax *has increased.*

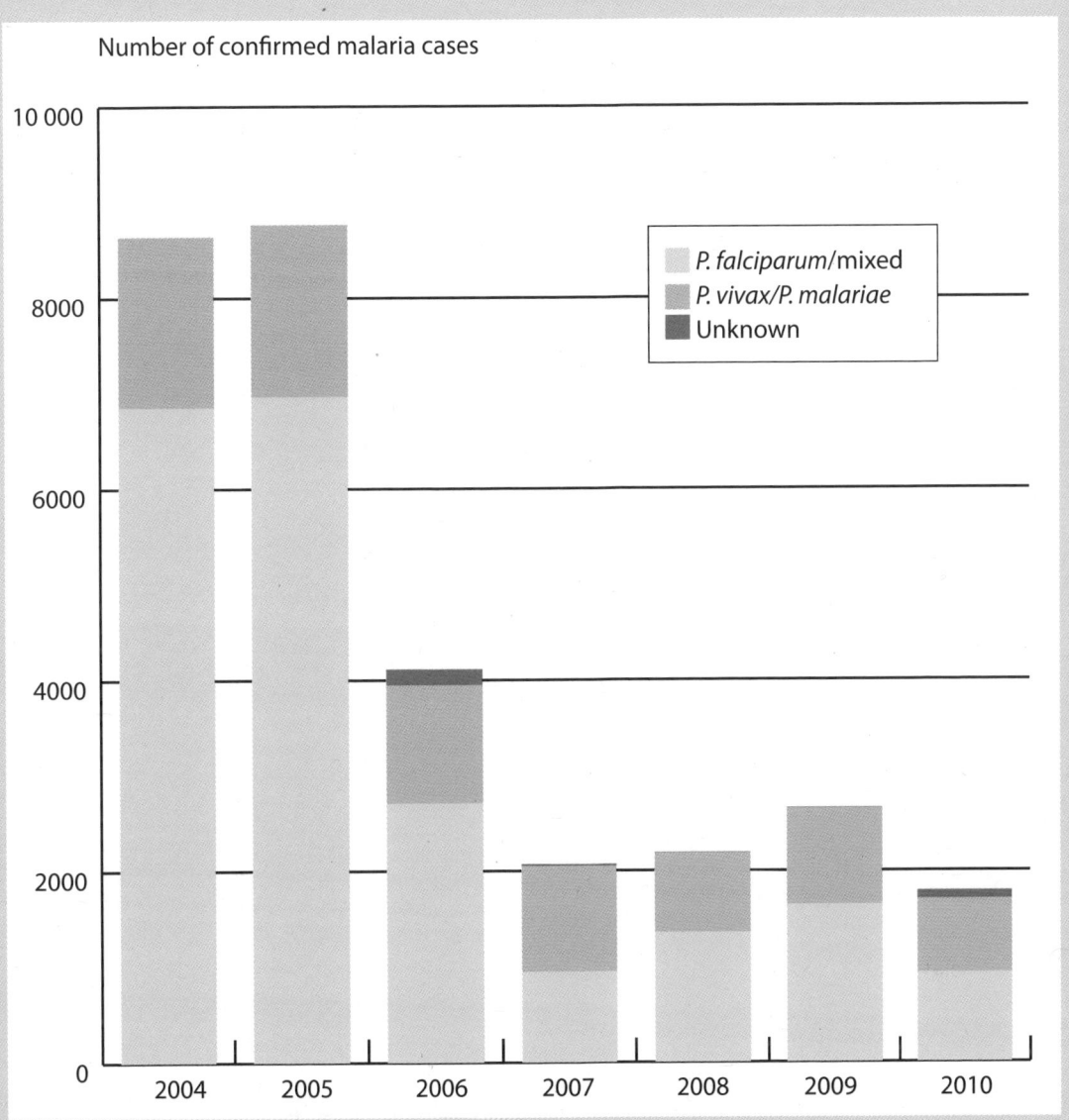

Note: Both local and imported cases are taken into account here.
Source: Ministry of Health Malaria Program in Suriname, 2011.

Box 5.1. Malaria control in Suriname (continued)

The Ministry of Health is responsible for malaria control. In communities in the interior of the country, services are provided by the Medical Mission, an NGO primarily financed by the government. The mobile gold mining communities, because of their illegal status and activities, often work in remote localities, out of reach of the Medical Mission health services.

The number of reported malaria cases in Suriname has decreased markedly from 11 361 in 2000 to 544 in 2010. The most significant decreases in cases occurred between 2005 and 2010, during which time malaria control activities were expanded with the support of a US$ 5 million grant of the Global Fund to Fight AIDS, Tuberculosis and Malaria. As cases of malaria in Suriname have decreased, the proportion due to *P. vivax* has increased (Figure 5.2).

The strategies adopted from 2005 included:

- Mass distribution of free long-lasting insecticidal nets.
- Indoor residual spraying in high risk areas.
- Strengthening of the case management system.
- Introduction of malaria service deliverers (MSDs) in remote areas.
- Active case detection (ACD) campaigns.
- A behaviour change communication programme.
- Strengthening of the epidemic detection and response system.
- Development of a new national malaria data collection tool and reporting system.

MSDs are used to reach the small-scale gold miners in remote areas. Members of the gold miner communities are selected and trained in providing malaria diagnosis by RDT and treatment to their fellow community members under the supervision of (and with quality assurance by) the malaria control programme. A new malaria diagnostic point was also established in the northern part of the capital of Suriname, a known gold miner trading locality. Health personnel at the diagnostic point are trained to provide malaria services to immigrants in their own language and disregard whether they were legal or illegal immigrants.

As the number of malaria cases decreased, the importance of malaria in gold miner communities increased. Initially most malaria cases were reported from both the new diagnostic point in the northern part of the capital and from ACD activities in gold mining areas. From 2009 onwards the Ministry of Health increased its emphasis on prevention and on ACD and MSD activities in mining areas with the support of US$ 5 million GF grant (round 7). An increasing proportion of the malaria cases found in the illegal immigrant gold miner communities appear to have been acquired in French Guiana and imported to Suriname as gold miners cross the border.

The Ministry of Health and National Malaria Board in Suriname has established a Malaria Control and Elimination Strategic Plan for the years 2011–2015 which ultimately aims to eliminate malaria by focused and scaled-up prevention and control activities in high-risk groups and areas. The development of a regional malaria control programme is necessary to reduce cross-border importation and close cooperation is sought with France and partnerships with malaria control authorities in French Guiana. The success of the plan will much depend on national and international commitment and support.

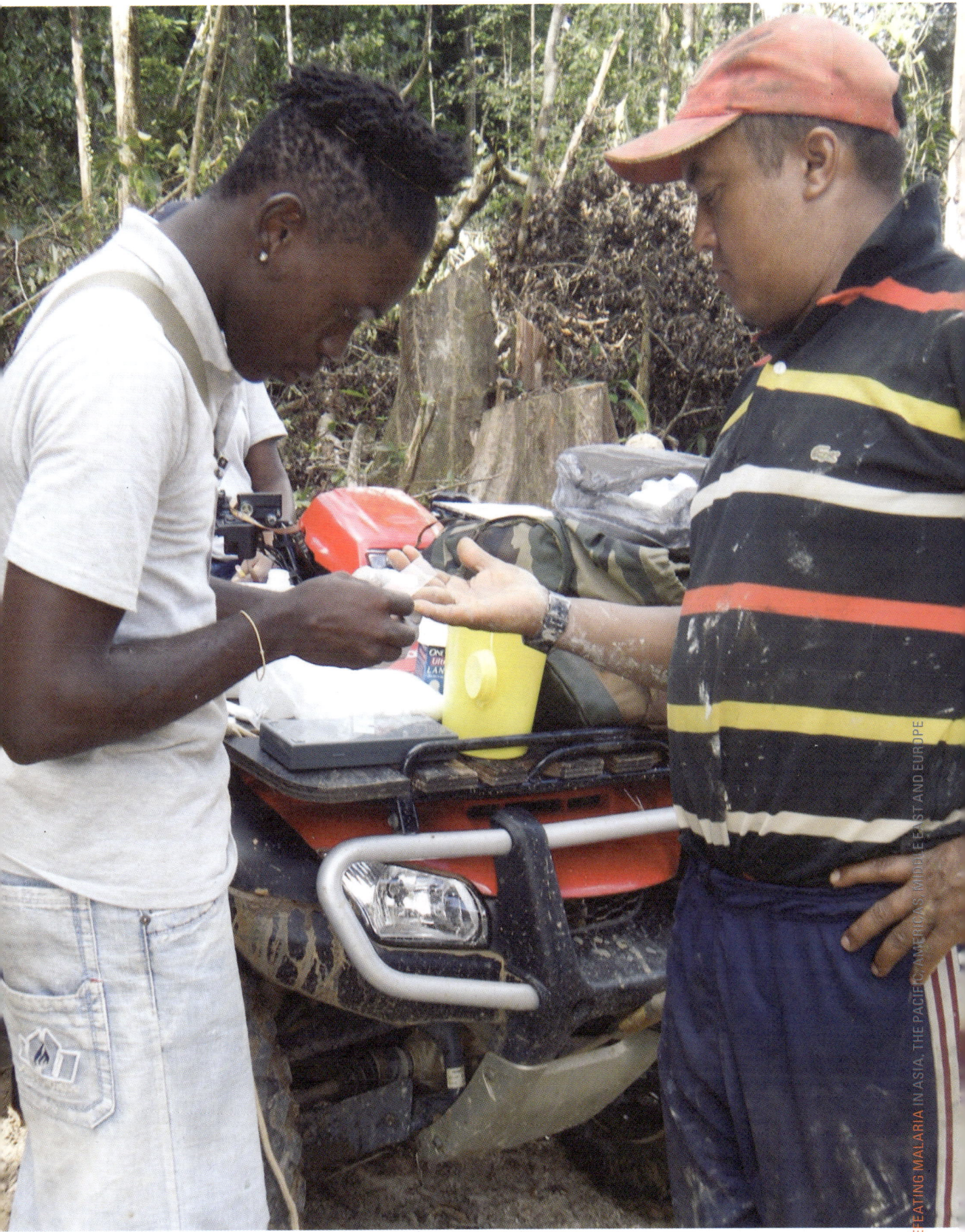

| THE AMERICAS |

Populations living in tropical rainforest areas of the Pacific coast of Colombia and Ecuador are also at significant risk of infection, particularly with *P. falciparum*. The majority of the population in these areas is of African descent and live in remote, hard to reach communities.

Hispaniola is the only island in the Caribbean where malaria is endemic. The majority of cases arise from Haiti, which reported approximately 84 000 confirmed cases in 2010. The Dominican Republic reported only 2500 cases, mostly from areas bordering Haiti. The risk of malaria in Haiti increased following a force 7 earthquake in January 2010 with many people living in camps with rudimentary drainage systems which provide favorable conditions for breeding of malaria vectors. However, active control measures appear to have averted a major epidemic.

People ages 5 to 49 years, or the most economically productive ages of life, constitute the majority of the diagnosed cases in the region. The age-sex distribution follows that of the population. Urban malaria is reported in Belize, Brazil, Colombia, the Dominican Republic, and Venezuela while indigenous populations in Brazil, Colombia, Guyana, Mexico, and Panama are noted as among specific groups that remain vulnerable to malaria infection. Cases of malaria among pregnant women are likewise reported in some areas of Bolivia, Brazil, Colombia, Guyana, Haiti, Panama, and Suriname.

Vectors

There are two principal vectors of malaria in the Americas, *An. albimanus* and *An. darlingi*. *An. albimanus* is the main vector in Central America and the Caribbean, extending north to Mexico and south to Ecuador. In the dry season, it is confined to coastal lagoons of brackish water but in the wet season it also breeds in small temporary rain pools inland. *An. albimanus* is often responsible for brief, highly localized outbreaks of *P. vivax* in Central America where only a small proportion of people get infected in any one year. It is an inefficient vector feeding largely on animals (zoophilic) and is not long lived. *An. albimanus* commonly rests outside and so is not a good target for IRS or ITNs, however, as it is a poor vector, even a limited impact from interventions can be effective at interrupting transmission.

An. darlingi is the main vector in the Amazon and Orinoco basins. It is a forest breeder, exploiting eddy-pools and very slow-moving water in small tributaries to larger rivers. The larvae are often found hiding among floating leaves. It has a high vectorial capacity, and because it is found principally in forests, IRS and ITNs are only partially effective for vector control.

Interventions

Microscopy is widely available and accessible and continues to be the primary method of diagnosis for malaria in the region. The availability and use of RDTs has increased since 2005. Belize, Costa Rica, Ecuador, and El Salvador report 100% of cases are diagnosed within 72 hours of onset of symptoms. The use of ACTs has increased gradually since 2005 (Box 5.2). No evidence exists of clinical failure of chloroquine treatment in persons with *P. falciparum* infection acquired in Hispaniola, nor has chloroquine prophylaxis failure been documented in travelers. Diagnosis and treatment is generally provided free of charge in all endemic countries.

Box 5.2: The Amazon Malaria Initiative

Launched in 2001, the Amazon Malaria Initiative (AMI) is a collaborative effort by the U.S. Agency for International Development Latin American and Caribbean Bureau and the Pan American Health Organization (PAHO). The rationale for creating AMI was and remains the need to invest in targeted activities to improve malaria control in Amazon Basin countries (Bolivia, Brazil, Colombia, Ecuador, Guyana, Peru, Surinam, and Venezuela) where 88% of malaria cases in Latin America and the Caribbean are reported. Through AMI, national malaria control programmes are able to share experiences and collaborate to address issues of common interest and concern. AMI's initial focus was to support the introduction of artemisinin-based combination therapies (ACTs) for *falciparum* malaria in all Amazon Basin countries and to improve access to malaria diagnosis and treatment (Figure 5.3).

Figure 5.3
Changes in policies for treatment of non-complicated *falciparum* malaria in AMI countries, 2000–2006

The Amazon Basin Initiative has been successful in improving member countries' national policies on access to ACTs, diagnostics, and treatment.

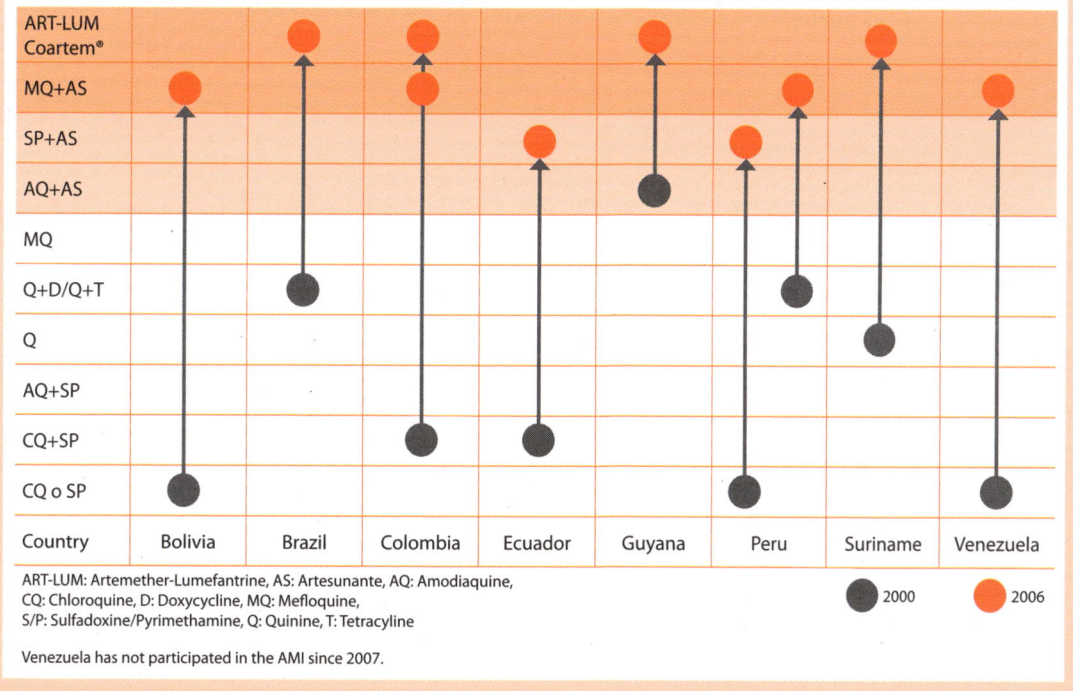

ART-LUM: Artemether-Lumefantrine, AS: Artesunante, AQ: Amodiaquine, CQ: Chloroquine, D: Doxycycline, MQ: Mefloquine, S/P: Sulfadoxine/Pyrimethamine, Q: Quinine, T: Tetracyline

Venezuela has not participated in the AMI since 2007.

Source: USAID and concerned NMCPs, 1995–2006.

| THE AMERICAS |

> **Box 5.2. The Amazon Malaria Initiative (continued)**
>
> AMI has been instrumental in helping countries implement ACT for laboratory-confirmed malaria cases and monitor efficacy. As a consequence the number of malaria cases treated with ACTs increased from zero in 2000 to 238 416 in 2009.
>
> AMI is now working on the following priority areas for the region: (1) Consolidating the gains achieved during the first 10 years of work, providing further attention to vivax malaria and to populations with special needs; (2) Making malaria control activities more sustainable, independently of AMI contribution; (3) Developing a regional approach to malaria prevention and control; (4) Helping national malaria control programmes be part of the decentralization effort in the health sector and adapting malaria control strategies to diverse and evolving epidemiological settings; and (5) Implementing the Strategy and Plan of Action for Malaria in the Americas for 2011–2015.

Both ITNs and IRS are used as preventive vector control measures against malaria. ITNs have been promoted since 2002 and LLINs since 2005. More than half a million nets have been distributed each year since 2005. IRS is used in most countries with 7.8 million people protected in 2009.

Domestic funding for malaria control has increased steadily since 2000 amounting to approximately US$ 190 million in 2009. It remains the primary source of funding for malaria control in the Americas. Total disbursements from the Global Fund for malaria control in 2010 were US$ 26.7 million.

Summary

The widespread decline in malaria cases and deaths in the Americas has resulted in considerable diversity in the status of control programmes within the region spanning the spectrum of prevention and control, pre-elimination, prevention of reintroduction, and complex emergencies. Despite much progress, significant challenges remain since populations with the highest incidence share several characteristics: they have limited access to services, limited infrastructure, extreme poverty, and settlements in hard to reach, scattered, rural areas or marginal urban areas. Developing and implementing programmes for these populations requires political commitment and appropriate levels of finance.

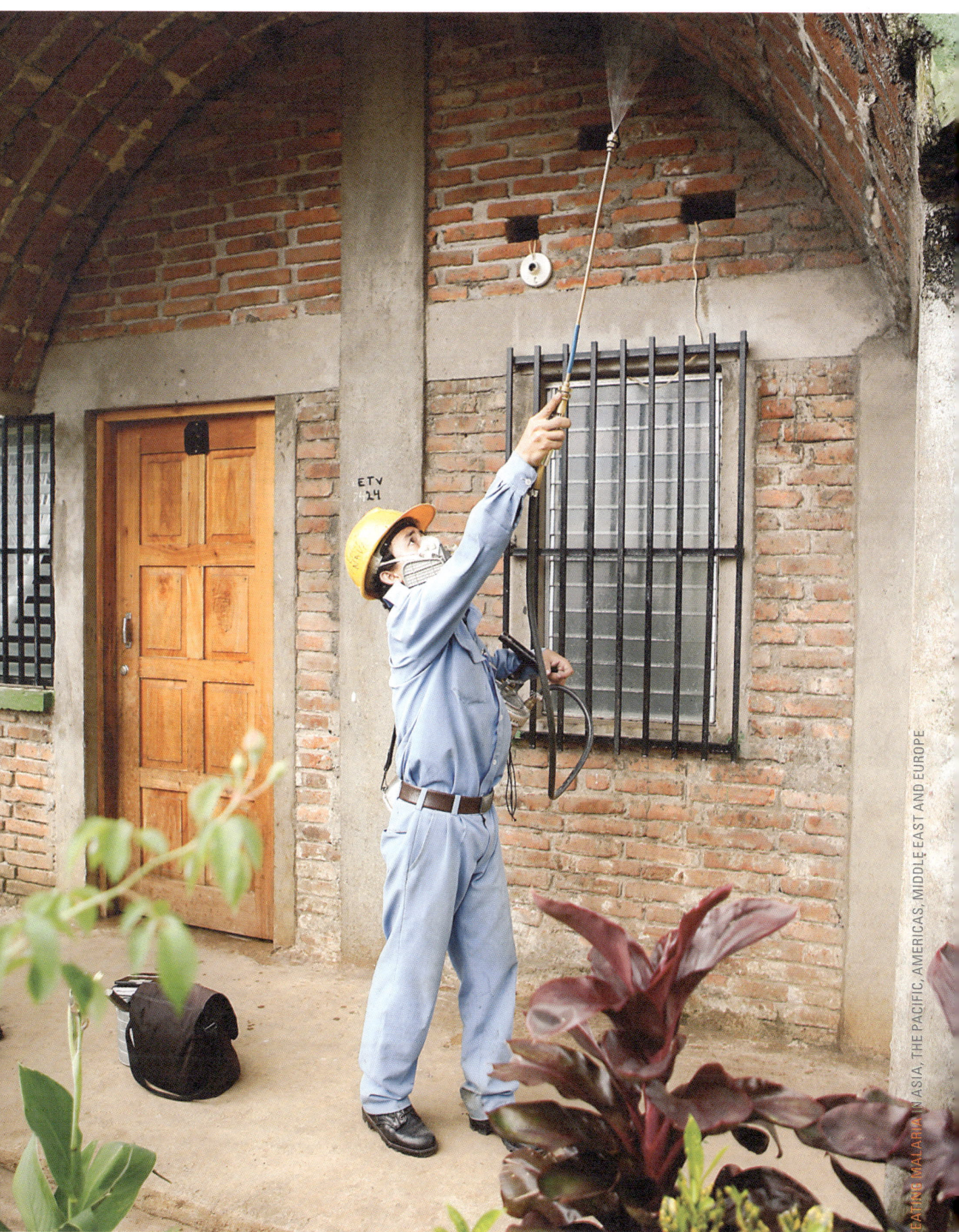

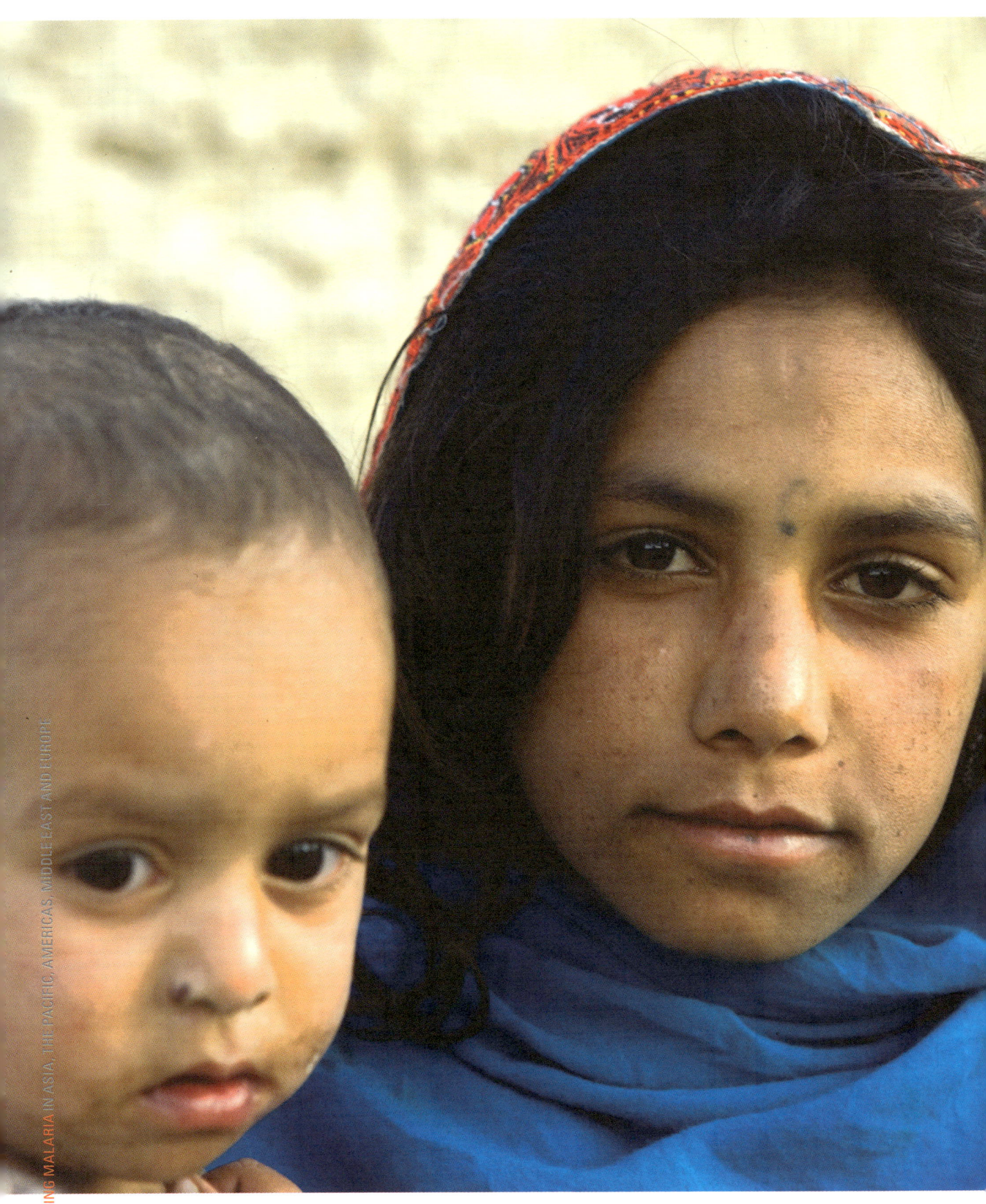

CHAPTER VI

THE ARABIAN PENINSULA, THE CAUCASUS AND NORTH-WEST ASIA

Nine countries in this region experienced ongoing malaria transmission in 2010, while two others reported zero locally acquired cases and one was certified as malaria-free. Afghanistan, Pakistan, and Yemen—which have relatively weak health systems—have areas of high malaria transmission, accounting for more than 95% of regional cases. The three highest-burden countries are particularly challenged by the magnitude of the problem and by security concerns; nevertheless, areas of each country have seen important progress in recent years.

Countries in control phase: Afghanistan, Pakistan, Yemen

Countries in pre-elimination phase: None

Countries in elimination phase: Azerbaijan, Iran, Kyrgyzstan, Saudi Arabia, Tajikistan, Turkey, Uzbekistan

Countries in prevention of reintroduction phase: Egypt, Georgia, Iraq, Oman, Russian Federation, Syrian Arab Republic

Population at risk: 250 million; 56% of the resident population

Parasitological species of reported malaria cases: P. falciparum 41%, P. vivax 59%, P. ovale, P. malariae

Main vectors: An. sacharovi, An. subpictus, An. sergentii, An. Arabiensis, An. culicifacies, An. siniensis

Estimated number of cases: 2.9 million; 1.3% of global total, 8.3% of total outside of Africa

Estimated number of malaria deaths: 3100; 0.5% of global total, 6.7% of total outside of Africa

Source: World Malaria Report 2011 (*16*).

| THE ARABIAN PENINSULA, THE CAUCASUS AND NORTH-WEST ASIA |

Epidemiological situation

In 2010 there were nine countries with ongoing transmission of malaria in this region (Afghanistan, Azerbaijan, Iran, Iraq, Kyrgyzstan, Pakistan, Saudi Arabia, Tajikistan, Turkey, Yemen). Armenia and Turkmenistan continue to report zero locally-acquired cases and Turkmenistan was certified as malaria-free in October 2010. Uzbekistan reported zero local cases for the first time in 2009, and Georgia and Iraq in 2010.

The region includes three countries with areas of high malaria transmission and relatively weak health systems (Afghanistan, Pakistan, and Yemen). These countries contribute more than 95% of reported cases in the region. The other 10 countries have low levels of malaria transmission and effective malaria programmes with ambitions to eliminate malaria from within their borders. *P. falciparum* is the dominant species of parasite in Saudi Arabia and Yemen, but *P. vivax* is more common in Afghanistan and Pakistan and accounts for almost all cases in Iran. Locally acquired malaria is entirely due to *P. vivax* in Azerbaijan, Kyrgyzstan, Tajikistan, and Turkey although imported cases of *P. falciparum* do occur (Map 6.1). In these countries, the number of remaining cases is small, but generally found in many small and geographically dispersed foci, presenting challenges to malaria elimination efforts.

Map 6.1

Proportion of cases due to *P. falciparum* in the Arabian Peninsula, the Caucasus, and North-West Asia, 2010

P. falciparum *is the dominant species of parasite in Saudi Arabia and Yemen, but* P. vivax *is more common in Afghanistan and Pakistan and accounts for almost all cases in Iran.*

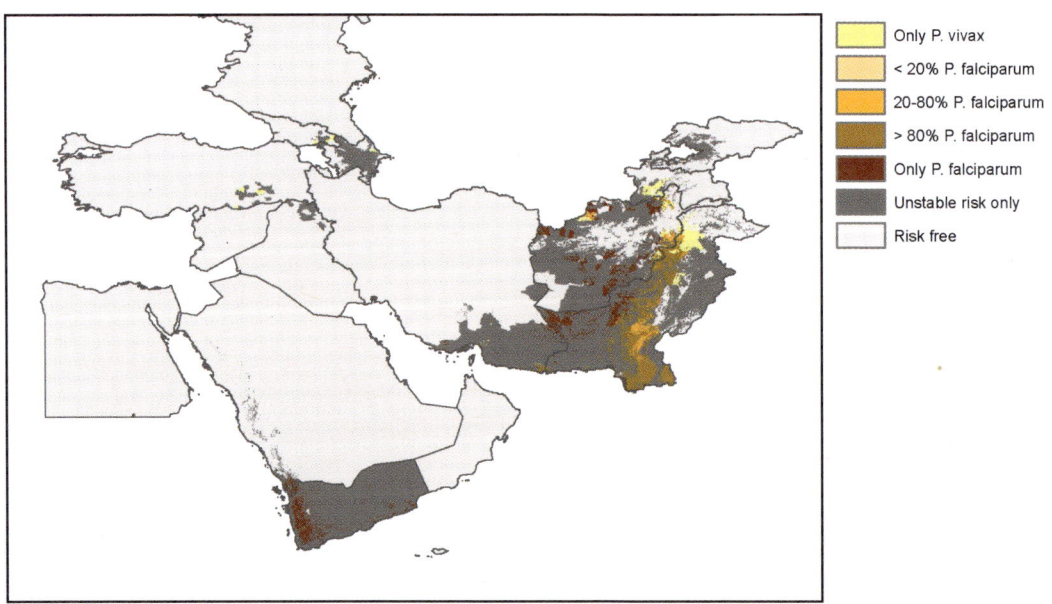

Note: Proportions are based on a four-year average of calculated annual parasite index for *P. falciparum* and *P. vivax* through 2010 and may not reflect the most recently reported subnational data.
Map production and source: Malaria Atlas Project (*17, 18*).

The reported number of cases in Pakistan and Yemen has remained stable over the past decade, although considerable progress in reducing the number of cases has been made in the Punjab, (Pakistan) and on Socotra Island (Yemen), which has no recorded local transmission of malaria since 2006. Afghanistan has reported a decrease in confirmed cases since 2002 against a background of increasing health service provisions (Figure 6.1a). The countries with the lowest levels of burden have shown immense progress in reducing the number of cases of malaria since 2000 (Figure 6.1b).

Figure 6.1
Trends in confirmed cases in the Arabian Peninsula, the Caucasus, and North-West Asia

(a) Countries with more than 30 000 reported confirmed cases in 2010. Note that the increase in cases in Pakistan in 2010, which affects the overall total, may be due to more patients receiving a diagnostic test rather than a real increase in the number of cases in the community.

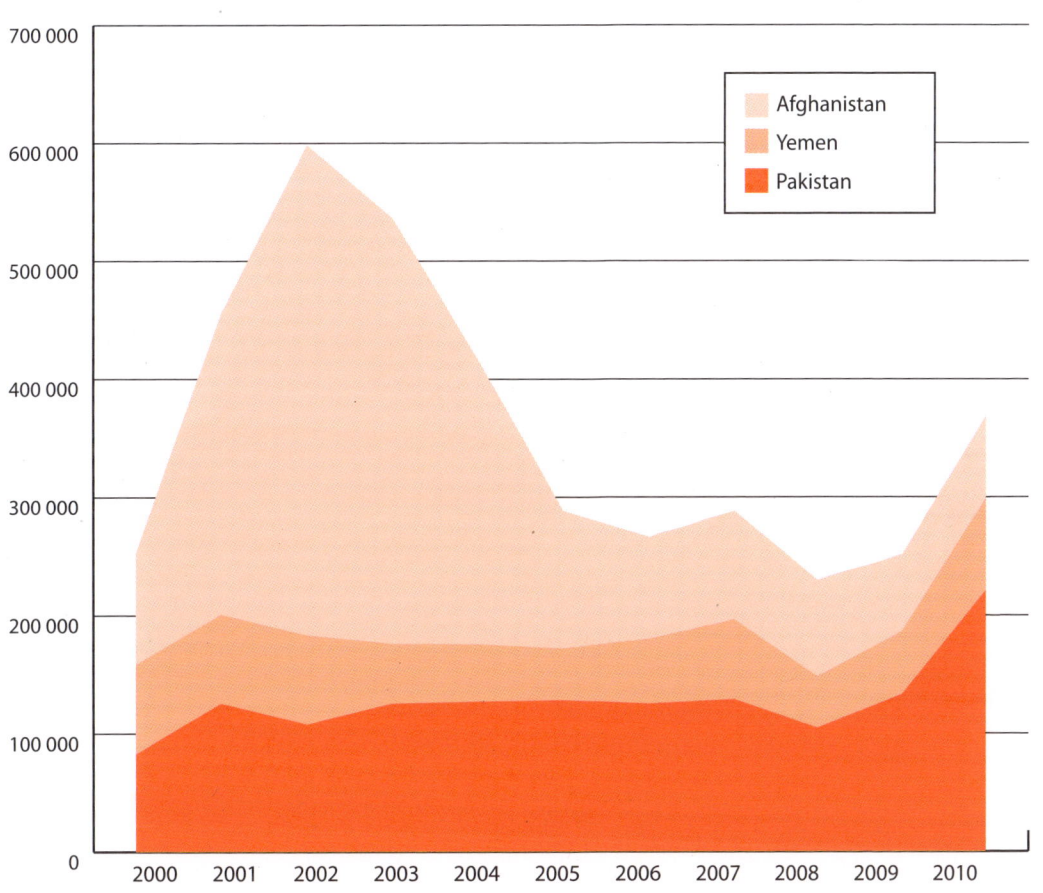

| THE ARABIAN PENINSULA, THE CAUCASUS AND NORTH-WEST ASIA |

(b) Countries with less than 30 000 reported confirmed cases in 2010. Countries with lower malaria burdens have shown tremendous progress in malaria cases.

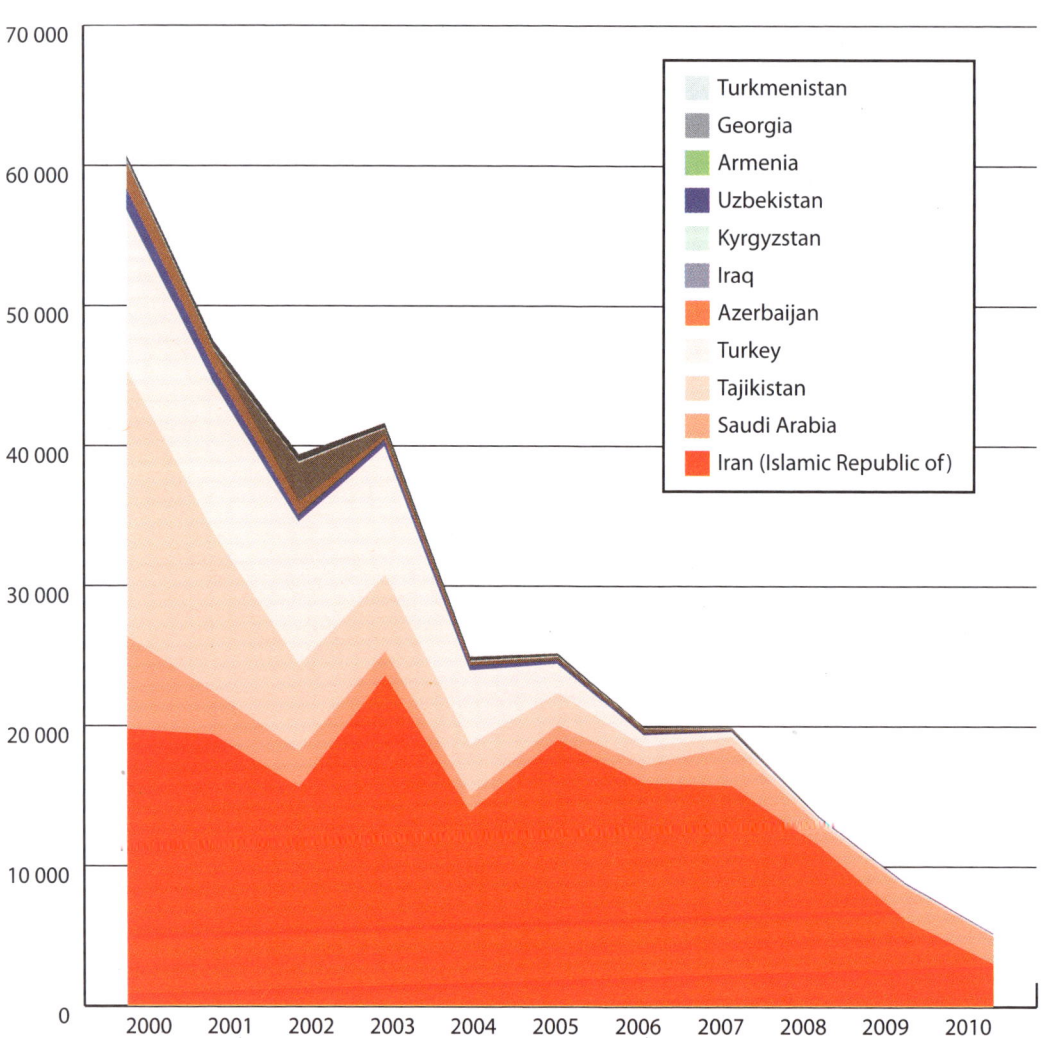

Source: World Malaria Report 2011 (*16*).

Populations affected
In all affected countries of this region, malaria transmission shows a marked focal distribution and is highly seasonal with most transmission occurring between June and November, although some transmission with *P. vivax* can occur earlier in the year. *P. falciparum* is unstable in this region, being at the edge of its range, and can fluctuate markedly from year to year depending on climatic variation. The seasonality and relatively low levels of transmission result in a population that is only partly immune to malaria; cases can occur in all age groups according to the degree of exposure (Figure 6.2).

Figure 6.2
Age-sex distribution of cases in Turkmenistan, 1999-2008

A large number of cases occurred in oil gas workers that worked in districts bordering Afghanistan and were infected by mosquitoes crossing the border, hence a peak in cases in males aged 20-29.

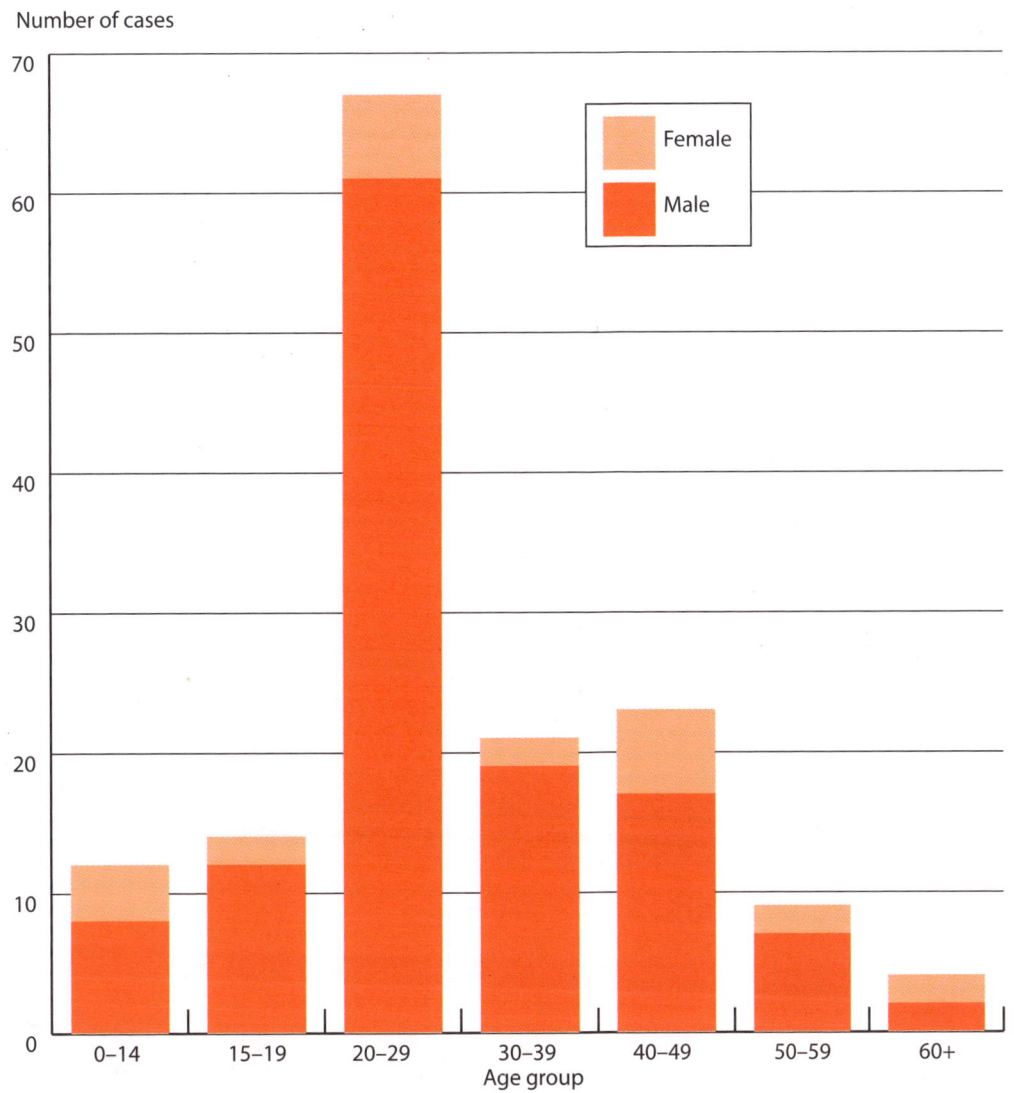

Source: Ministry of Health Turkmenistan.

THE ARABIAN PENINSULA, THE CAUCASUS AND NORTH-WEST ASIA

Vectors

Countries in the north-west of the region have a dry climate that supports *An. sacharovi* and *An. subpictus* as the primary vectors. *An. sacharovi* is indoor resting and biting and hibernates over the winter months although it may feed intermittently (*34*). Further east and south in Iran, Iraq, Saudi Arabia, and Yemen, dryness increases with desert interspersed with fertile river valleys. Here the primary vector is *An. sergentii*, which has mixed biting and resting habits (*36*), or, in Saudi Arabia and the mainland of Yemen, *An. arabiensis*, which breeds in temporary pools. To the north and east into Afghanistan, with high elevations and latitudes, the vector changes to more Asian species, notably *An. culicifacies* and *An. siniensis*. None of the vectors are considered to be particularly efficient transmitters of malaria.

Interventions

Countries within the WHO European Region (Azerbaijan, Georgia, Kyrgyzstan, Tajikistan, Turkey) signed the Tashkent Declaration in 2005, the goal of which is to interrupt malaria transmission and eliminate the disease by 2015. Here IRS is the primary means of vector control, while larvivorous *Gambusia* fish are used to control mosquito larvae in rice-growing areas. ITNs are used for protection in Tajikistan. All suspected cases of malaria are parasitologically tested and treated; information on the origins of each case is also gathered to determine if it is locally transmitted or imported.

IRS is also the main form of vector control in Saudi Arabia and Pakistan. ITNs are more commonly used in Afghanistan and Yemen. Parasitological testing of suspected cases is universal in Iran, Iraq, and Saudi Arabia but less common in Afghanistan, Pakistan, and Yemen where 62%, 60%, and 89% of suspected cases receive a parasitological test, respectively. Iran undertakes active case detection in its efforts to achieve elimination.

Control efforts are constrained by security concerns in a number of countries in this region. However, malaria control activities have continued amid some of the most challenging circumstances in Afghanistan, Iraq, and the Federally Administered Tribal Areas of Pakistan. In Afghanistan progress has been made by involving local and international NGOs in the distribution of ITNs (Box 6.1).

Summary

The region has witnessed considerable success in reducing the incidence of malaria in countries with the lowest burdens and the target of eliminating malaria from the WHO European Region by 2015 appears achievable. Control of malaria is more challenging in countries with higher burdens (Afghanistan, Pakistan, and Yemen) partly because the size of the problem is bigger but also, in places, because of security concerns. Despite these challenges progress has been made in some areas of the higher burden countries since 2000.

Box 6.1: Delivering ITNs in Afghanistan

Malaria is endemic in many parts of Afghanistan below 2000 metres, particularly in river valleys used for rice cultivation. Three epidemiological strata are recognized: (1) high-risk provinces (14 provinces, 12.5 million people), (2) low-risk provinces (15 provinces, 9.5 million people), and (3) very low risk or malaria-free provinces (5 provinces, 2.5 million people).

Map 6.2
Location of high, low, and very low risk provinces in Afghanistan

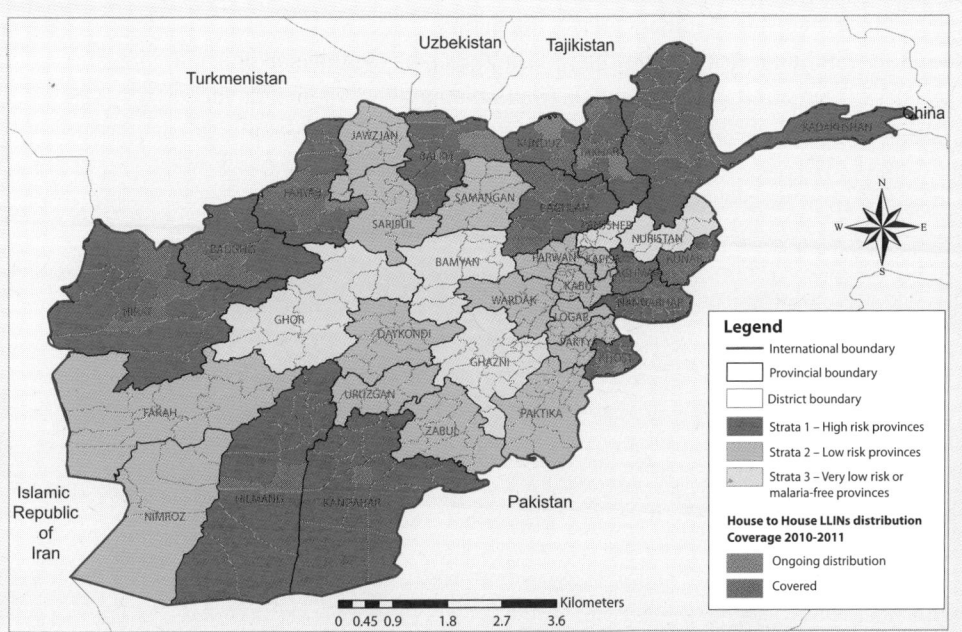

Source: HealthNet TPO and WHO Afghanistan, 2012.
Map production: MCE Data management, WHO Afghanistan.

Vector control lies at the heart of malaria control efforts in Afghanistan. The National Malaria and Leishmaniasis Control Programme (NMLCP) prioritizes the procurement, free supply, and proper utilization of long-lasting insecticidal nets (LLINs) in its efforts to secure universal access to vector control. Distributing LLINs in Afghanistan has never been an easy undertaking. The terrain is mountainous, communities are widely spread, and there is a lack of road infrastructure at every level. Extreme heat in the summer and heavy snowfalls in the winter also create challenges for storing and distributing LLINs. The supply of LLINs to some areas is also affected by security conditions which pose a direct threat to distribution personnel and bednets.

To overcome these challenges, the NMLCP works closely with international and local NGOs which are coordinated by HealthNet TPO. This organization commenced operations in Afghanistan in 1995, when conventional ITNs were distributed on a very small scale through a pilot project in a few provinces. The strategies for distributing ITNs have evolved over time, progressively achieving higher levels of coverage:

| THE ARABIAN PENINSULA, THE CAUCASUS AND NORTH-WEST ASIA |

Box 6.1. Delivering ITNs in Afghanistan (continued)

Social marketing: ITNs were initially distributed by selling them at highly subsidized prices by district clinics and mobile teams of educators and salesmen in more remote areas. ITNs were also distributed to parents of children who came to routine vaccination clinics.

Social marketing plus free distribution through clinics: In 2005, LLINs were introduced and distributed free of charge to pregnant women and children under five years of age attending antenatal care (ANC) clinics and DPT3 vaccinations respectively, with support from the Global Fund. Sales at highly subsidized prices also continued for other population groups. In 2009, under the provision in the Afghanistan Constitution for free health care services, social marketing of LLINs was discontinued and LLINs were distributed only free of charge through ANC clinics and at DPT3 vaccination.

Household distribution: In 2008 access to LLINs was greatly expanded by providing them to households in high-risk provinces through house-to-house distribution. Standard operating procedures were developed for the proper storage and distribution of LLINs and were adopted at all supply points. Distribution teams, each consisting of one project manager, two ITN officers, and one supplier, were established in all 14 high risk provinces. A pre-distribution census was conducted by community health workers with the support of community and religious leaders. During the registration and listing of households, vouchers were distributed which indicated the number of LLINs that each household was entitled to. LLINs were then distributed through a distribution point within each village against the vouchers. While the strategy has greatly expanded access to LLINs, it has not been without difficulties; for example, delays in procurement and supply of LLINs resulted in stock-outs of LLINs for several months.

The expansion of LLIN coverage in high risk provinces benefited from Round 8 Global Fund support. Additional resources will be required to ensure the replacement of LLINs after they reach their recommended life span. After attaining high coverage in high risk provinces, emphasis will be placed on achieving and maintaining high coverage of vulnerable groups and key affected populations in low risk provinces.

Figure 6.3
Increasing numbers of ITNs distributed in Afghanistan

2007 marked the beginning of an era of increased ITN distribution in Afghanistan.

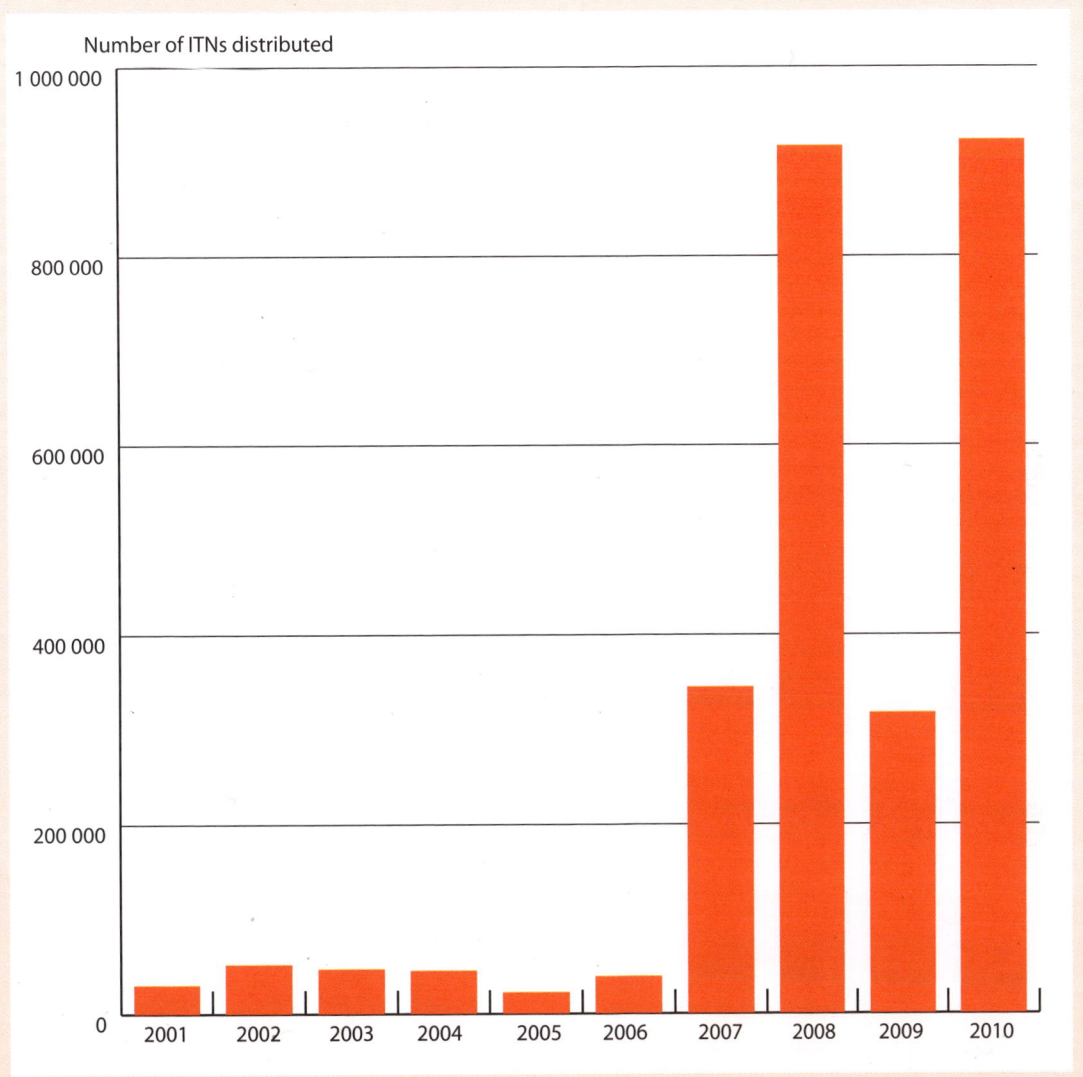

Source: National Malaria and Leishmaniasis Control Programme (NMLCP) and HealthNet TPO.

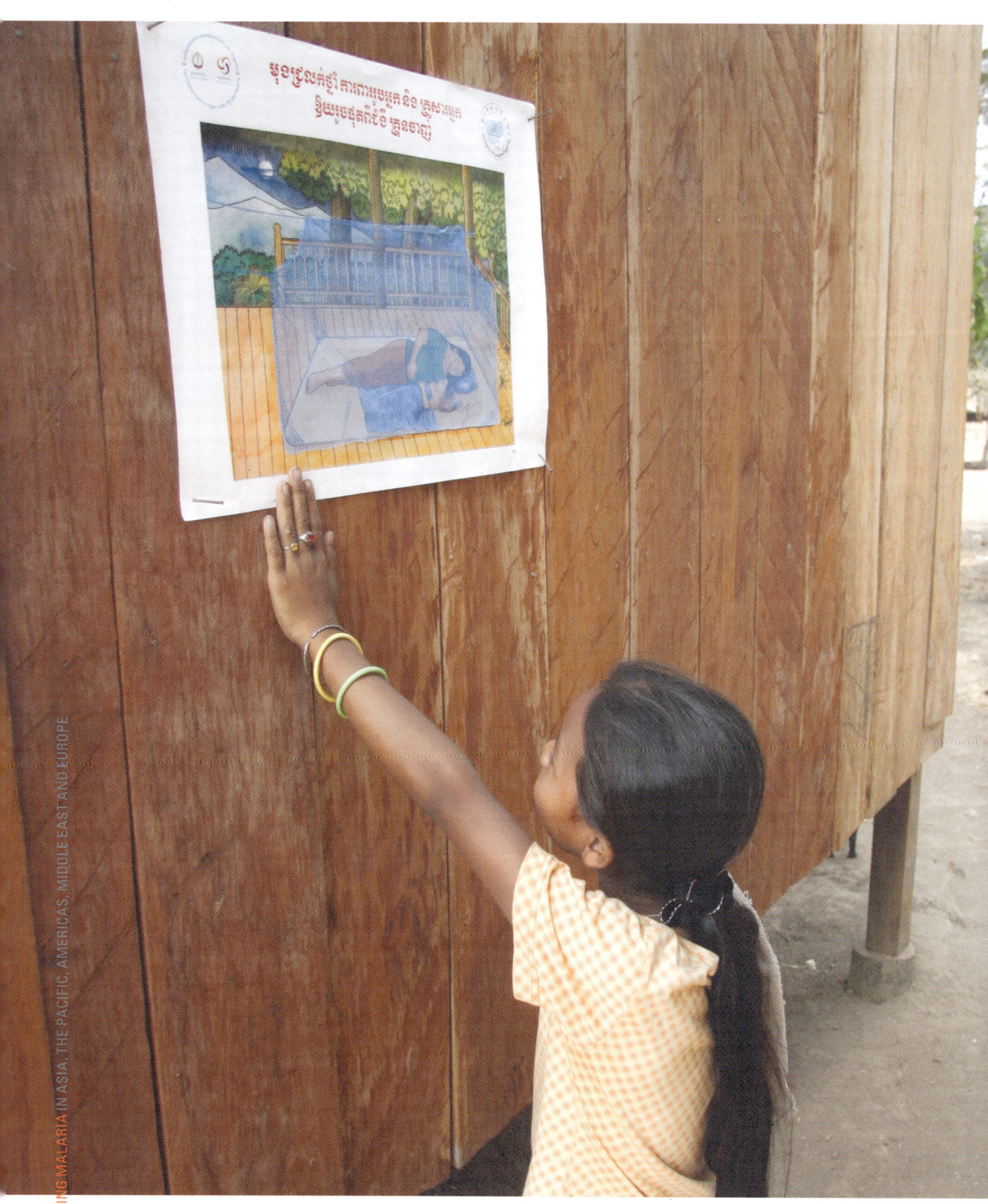

CHAPTER VII

REDUCING MALARIA BRINGS SUCCESS AND NEW CHALLENGES

While there are many successes to celebrate, this has brought about important changes. The shrinking of the malaria map outside of Africa is an important success that provides strong foundations for additional progress. At the same time, this means that while some population sub-groups are now at reduced risk, the disease is becoming increasingly concentrated in marginalized populations. As P. falciparum *is controlled,* P. vivax, *and its unique challenges, may become more prominent. Proactively anticipating and addressing these challenges is critical. Diluting or disrupting national commitment to malaria control likely will lead to malaria resurgence.*

The preceding sections of this report illustrate the heterogeneity of malaria epidemiology across the world and the success with which some countries have controlled the disease. As malaria transmission declines, several changes become apparent:

The malaria map in the region is shrinking, with strong potential for additional progress. Several countries are now on the brink of elimination; four countries have been certified as free of malaria since 2007 (Armenia, Morocco, Turkmenistan, and the United Arab Emirates). The WHO European Region is aiming to eliminate malaria across the entire region by 2015. *P. falciparum* transmission has already been eliminated from the region, with the last cases reported in Tajikistan in 2008. Georgia reported zero locally-acquired cases in 2010. Only Azerbaijan (50 cases in 2010), Tajikistan (111 cases), and Turkey (9 cases) still report local *P. vivax* malaria transmission. Argentina, El Salvador, Mexico, and Paraguay have reported few malaria cases (mostly *P. vivax*) in recent years. Iraq reported no cases arising from local transmission in 2009 and 2010. Bhutan reported only 401 cases in 2010, while Sri Lanka has reduced the number of cases from more than 200 000 in 2000 to less than 700 in 2010. Several other countries are adopting strategies to eliminate malaria.

Different population sub-groups are at greatest risk of malaria infection. When malaria transmission decreases, little immunity is developed in childhood and malaria can occur in any age group according to the degree of prior exposure. Thus, among forest workers in Viet Nam, Cambodia, and Brazil (who often originate from areas with no malaria), adult males are at greatest risk of the disease. For these populations, ITNs in the home may offer little protection since infections are mostly acquired when sleeping in the forest; instead, forest workers may benefit from insecticide-treated hammocks which can be used in the forest and from diagnostic and treatment facilities near their workplaces.

REDUCING MALARIA BRINGS SUCCESS AND NEW CHALLENGES

Malaria becomes increasingly concentrated in marginalized populations. Ethnic, religious, and political minorities may have a high burden of malaria despite good control within the general population. For example, in India although tribal communities constitute only 8% of the total population of the country, they contribute 25% of the total malaria cases. This may be due to the geography of where marginalized populations live, such as mountainous areas that are difficult to access, but also because ethnic minorities may find access to formal health care and preventive measures difficult due to language, traditional beliefs, and health-seeking behaviours.

Malaria transmission intensity can be highly heterogeneous within countries. While some populations may be at reduced risk of malaria others may be subject to high incidence. Malaria control programmes therefore need to take into account the circumstances of specific risk groups or specific geographic areas to develop appropriate strategies to control malaria.

Migration becomes an increasingly important concern. Where there is considerable heterogeneity in the intensity of malaria transmission, migration of people from non-endemic or low transmission areas to endemic or high transmission areas or vice versa becomes a much more prominent issue for malaria control programmes. Migrant populations coming from non-endemic areas have not developed immunity to malaria and can easily become sick when working in an endemic area. Examples include those working in the gold and gem mines in the Brazilian Amazon, forest workers in Cambodia, and refugees fleeing violence in Afghanistan or natural disasters in Sri Lanka. Their vulnerability to malaria infections may also be greater than that of local populations due to poor or absent housing, malnutrition, and other concurrent infections.

Migrants from endemic areas to less endemic areas may also present significant challenges to a malaria control programme particularly for countries or areas that are in the pre-elimination, elimination, and prevention of reintroduction phases of malaria control. In Oman, since 2007 there have been sporadic outbreaks of both

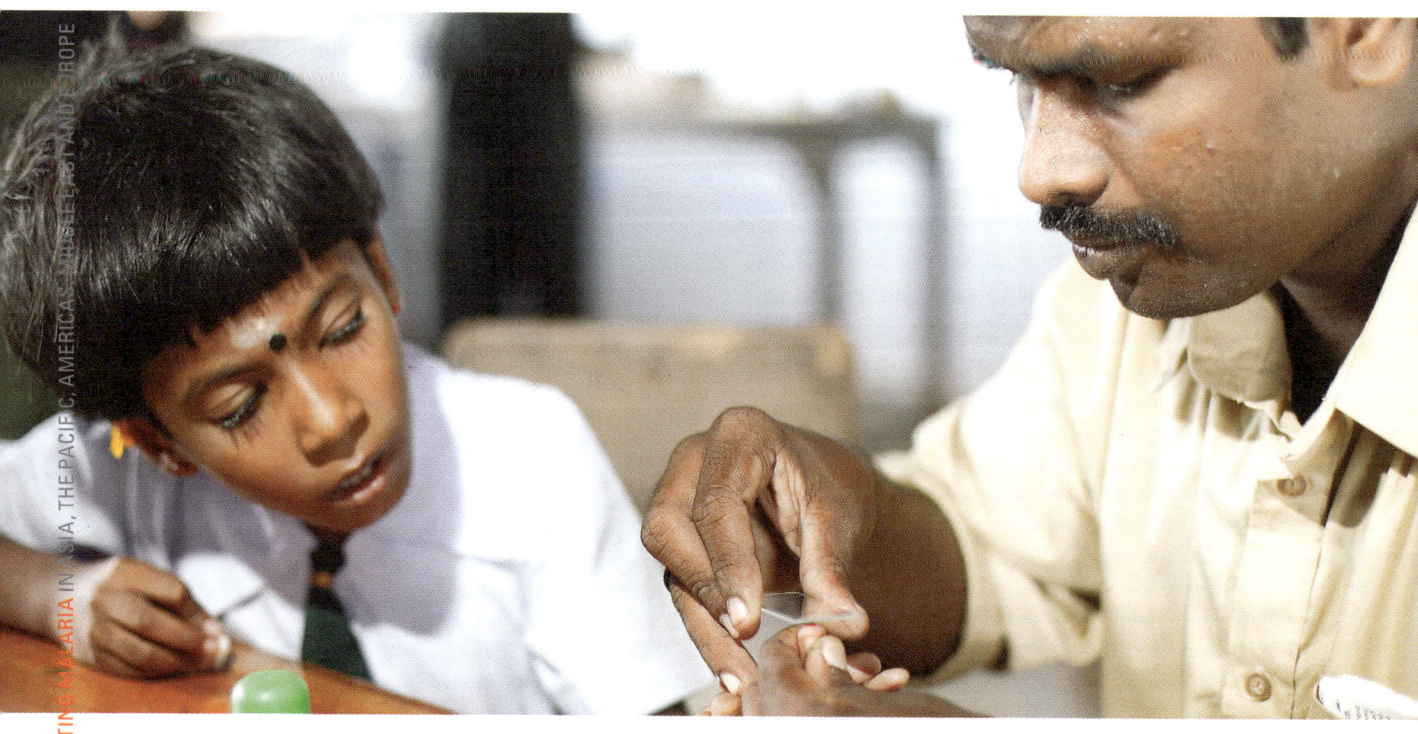

P. falciparum and *P. vivax* cases due to importation of infections from the Indian subcontinent. Singapore is prone to infections from travellers and small-scale outbreaks regularly occur and need to be controlled promptly.

Malaria is often focused on border areas. International borders are frequently defined by natural barriers with difficult terrain such mountains, valleys, and dense forests. Border regions are also often the least developed areas in a country and are populated by the poor who generally have the highest incidence of malaria. Sometimes the people living on either side of international borders have close ethnic and family ties resulting in frequent population movements across boundaries. For all of these reasons—in addition to security or political concerns—it may be difficult to offer services to populations living at national borders.

***P. vivax* may become increasingly important.** As malaria control is intensified, the number of cases due to *P. falciparum* falls more quickly than those of *P. vivax* so the proportion of cases due to *P. vivax* increases. Although *P. vivax* infections are less likely to lead to severe malaria and death, the parasite is tolerant of a wider range of environmental conditions, and so is more geographically widespread. It is also more difficult to control since it has a dormant liver stage which allows it to persist longer periods even if mosquitoes are not present for its transmission. The liver stage parasites cannot be detected with existing diagnostic tests and can only be eliminated by administering primaquine, which must be taken daily over 14 days. Unfortunately, primaquine can produce serious side-effects (hemolytic anaemia) in patients who have more severe forms of glucose-6-phosphate dehydrogenase (G6PD) deficiency. Testing for G6PD deficiency is currently technically challenging and relatively expensive, hence, many clinicians will not prescribe primaquine when the risk from the drug may exceed that from the disease. The development of a low-cost and accurate rapid diagnostic test for G6PD deficiency would be an important advance for the control of *vivax* malaria.

Malaria is apt to return if control measures are diluted or disrupted. As the incidence of malaria is reduced, naturally acquired immunity to the disease (which is at best partial) decreases. Although new infections are less likely to occur they can rapidly lead to illness, which can be severe, and they can more easily spread from one person to another. If control programmes are not maintained, devastating outbreaks or epidemics can occur (Box 7.1). Loss of political will as well as social and political unrest and natural calamities represent additional risks for epidemics. Increased vigilance and intensification of control efforts have prevented large-scale outbreaks following earthquakes in Haiti, the tsunami in Indonesia, flooding in Pakistan, and war situations such as Afghanistan's. The vast majority of resurgences in the past 80 years (91%) have been due, at least in part, to the weakening of malaria control programmes with resource constraints being the most commonly identified factor (57%) (*37*). Given that most malaria resurgences are linked to weakening of control programmes, a high level of commitment is needed to maintain control programmes even once success has been achieved.

Box 7.1: Outbreaks and epidemics

The concept of malaria outbreaks or epidemics has long been part of the language that we have used. It is a description applied to malaria when the incidence of cases (other than seasonal increases) in an area rises rapidly and markedly above its usual level or when the infection occurs in an area where it was not previously present (*38*).

However, in the context of marked progress in malaria control in a relatively short time frame, the concept of epidemics and outbreaks takes on a new face. This includes:

1. As transmission is reduced over a number of years, the population tends to loose immunity. On the one hand this is good as it means that most infections will rapidly lead to illness and, assuming that these cases present to the health workers, they can be rapidly treated and transmission can be curtailed. However, if a rapid response to illness and good services are not in place, such cases can go untreated and lead to severe disease. And, if conducive climatic conditions lead to higher vector populations and survival, the return of transmission can lead to many cases and fatalities—an epidemic.

2. As transmission is reduced to very low levels, individual cases of malaria become important as indicators of location and determinants of transmission risk—in essence an individual case becomes an outbreak.

3. Disruption or dilution of services (through loss of political will, local conflict, war, or environmental disasters) can also allow for the return of transmission and a major upsurge of cases and severe disease.

The preparation for these events is less and less about epidemic preparedness but, rather, the recognition that prevention of epidemics and outbreaks (even single cases) relies on continuation of control efforts (even in the absence of cases) and on enhanced vigilance so that cases are rapidly detected should they arise. If these are not undertaken, then the risk of return of transmission and consequent return of illness and severe disease will be rapid. All of this is predictable and preventable.

CHAPTER VIII

MALARIA PROGRAMME RESPONSE TO NEW CHALLENGES

The challenges discussed in Chapter 7 have a range of implications for malaria control programme design. As the specific needs of the most-affected populations change, countries must be adaptive and responsive. Malaria control programmes require detailed surveillance information focusing on parasitologically confirmed cases to ensure that appropriate prevention and treatment strategies are in place. Programmes must be alert to the possibility of epidemics while also monitoring the risk of drug and insecticide resistance. Instituting cross-border collaborations and shared learning between regions and countries is integral to overall success.

The challenges discussed in Chapter 7 have a range of implications for malaria control programme design.

Malaria programmes need to be adapted to the specific needs of populations most affected. The populations most at risk may be young children, adult males, ethnic minorities, or migrant populations. The range of services offered may also need to be more diverse, since malaria epidemiology may vary within a country resulting in high transmission areas adjacent to low transmission settings and areas that have eliminated malaria. In order to ensure that all people with malaria have access to high quality services, it will often be necessary to work with private sector providers to guarantee compliance with national guidelines for malaria diagnosis and treatment. It will also be necessary to develop and manage community-based programmes in areas where access to formal services is lacking. Where malaria is limited geographically, and in frequency, the management of programmes may need to be more vertical than in settings where malaria accounts for a high proportion of outpatient attendances and admissions and where malaria must be incorporated in the activities of all personnel working in a health system.

Malaria control programmes require detailed surveillance information to design appropriate strategies for prevention and treatment. Information is required on the populations most affected (such as where the disease occurs and in what age groups, sex, occupations, and ethnic groups), where infections are acquired (at home or elsewhere), vector behaviour (where and when they bite and rest), and the parasite involved (whether it is *P. vivax*, *P. falciparum*, or other species). When the distribution of malaria is patchy, and malaria infections are comparatively rare, nationally representative household surveys are unlikely to provide the required information

| MALARIA PROGRAMME RESPONSE TO NEW CHALLENGES |

for programme design. Rather, malaria control programme managers must utilize information from routine disease surveillance, monitoring, and evaluation systems and targeted operational research. In this situation, a programme may be largely reliant on surveillance as a first line of attack on the disease rather than the implementation of IRS or ITN programmes on a large scale. When levels of transmission are very low or in areas of elimination, every case needs to be investigated to determine whether it is imported or locally acquired and whether or not vector control measures need to be heightened. When malaria is confined to certain localities in a country, or is a relatively rare occurrence, extensive nationwide reporting through a general HMIS may not be justified and malaria control programmes may benefit from malaria-specific surveillance systems that can generate additional information on the population groups most affected (in contrast to settings where malaria accounts for the bulk of attendances at health facilities and national health information systems must incorporate malaria concerns). However, as malaria disappears and malaria surveillance-specific systems are no longer justifiable, they must be reintegrated into general communicable disease surveillance systems.

Surveillance systems need to focus on parasitologically confirmed cases by either microscopy or RDT. This is because a smaller proportion of fevers in low-prevalence settings are attributable to malaria, and it is important to know if infections are due to *P. falciparum* or *P. vivax* for guiding treatment response, estimating drug supply needs, and other planning purposes. In addition, given that a high proportion of cases may be treated by private sector providers, and the unsuitability of household surveys in many circumstances, it will be beneficial to establish mechanisms to obtain timely information from private sector providers and community-based programmes in order to establish a complete and evolving picture to monitor progress in malaria control.

Programmes must be alert to the possibility of epidemics. In areas where malaria transmission has been reduced by control measures but vectors are still abundant, control programmes need to be alert to the possibilities of resurgences and will need strong surveillance systems. Control efforts should continue even in the absence of cases and programmes need to be vigilant so that cases are rapidly detected and appropriately treated should they arise.

Drug and insecticide resistance monitoring will need to adapt with changing programme conditions. The development of drug and insecticide resistance represents a major threat to the effectiveness of existing interventions; however, resistance can be identified early, tracked appropriately, and changes can be introduced to manage the evolution of this resistance. Each country, with technical support from WHO and other partners, is responsible for monitoring its antimalarial drug resistance patterns. But detecting it is increasingly challenging because as malaria disappears it becomes more and more difficult to enroll enough infected patients to test drug efficacy using standard protocols, which require a minimum of fifty malaria patients at a sentinel site and testing at least every two years. It may be necessary to lower parasite thresholds for those patients included in studies, undertake efficacy testing less frequently than every two years, or combine results from different sites or different countries. As a practical measure, for areas where drug resistance has been reported, the number of patients who remain parasite positive after three days of treatment may be used as an indirect marker of artesunate resistance as on the Cambodia-Thailand border.

Cross-border collaborations. In areas where malaria is increasingly confined to border areas, cross-border communication and regional collaborations are important in order to develop joint solutions to common problems. Such collaborations can share data, share experience of successful strategies, develop regional plans,

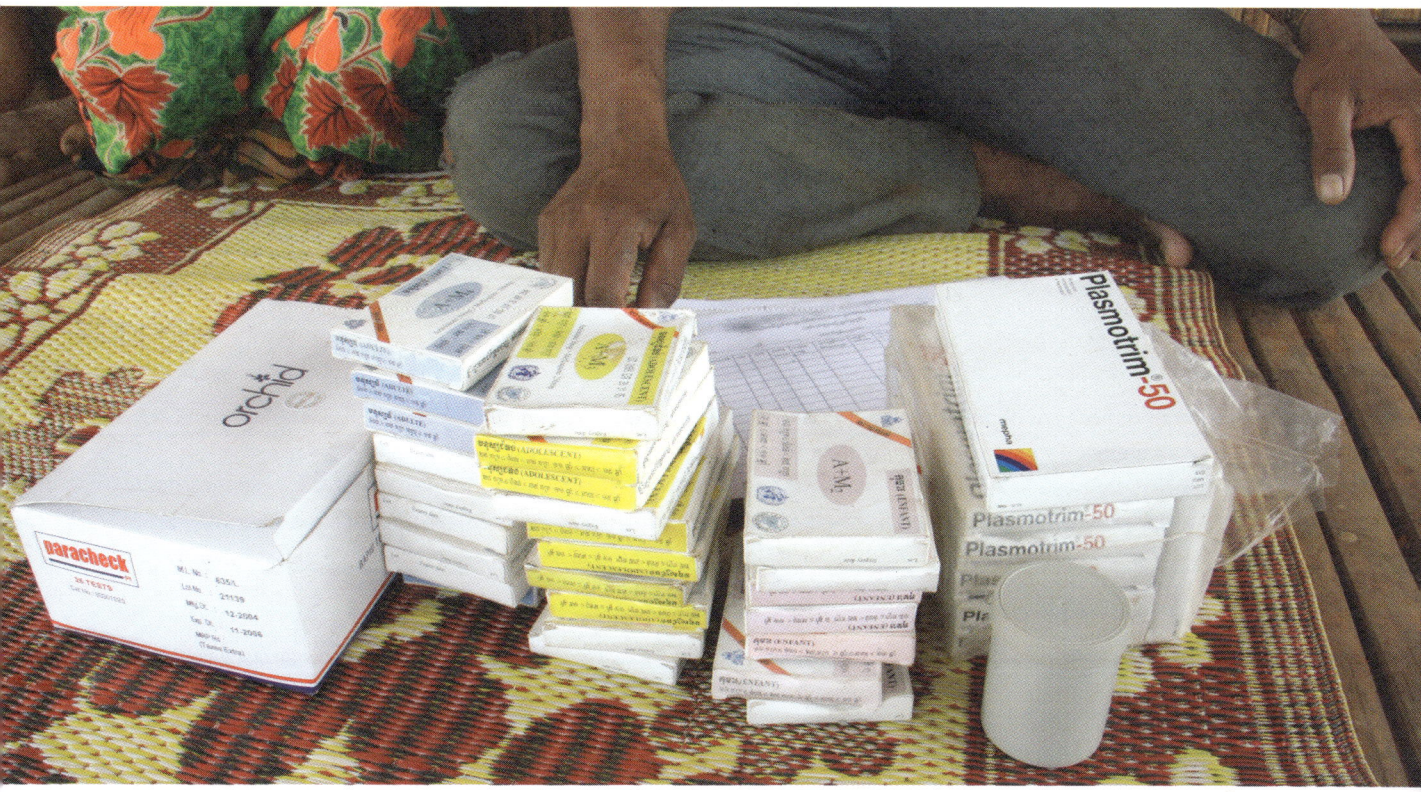

and conduct joint activities. Several strong collaborations are under way in a range of settings, establishing promising practices for success (Boxes 3.4, 4.2, and 5.2). These types of collaborations are particularly important where migration across borders represents a major source of new malaria infection. Senior managers and politicians will need to show leadership and creativity to develop cross-border relationships and strategies that are inclusive of marginalized populations.

Learning between regions and countries will be increasingly important in the coming years. The WHO European Region has embarked on elimination for all the countries with remaining malaria transmission; their successes and challenges will be instructive for other regions and countries, particularly outside of Africa. Malaria elimination for many countries in the Americas also appears to be a near-term opportunity; and each of the regions has several or many countries that could achieve elimination in the coming decade. Examining the implications for programme design and action noted above will be important as each country attempts—and hopefully achieves—elimination. Programme responses outlined here apply not just to countries in Asia, the Pacific, Americas, Middle East, and Europe but also to those in Africa. Attention to domestic political and financial commitment; the need to build information systems and surveillance early and to move completely to identifying, treating, and tracking confirmed malaria (not just suspected malaria); the need to track and respond to insecticide and drug resistance; and increasing attention to the smaller and smaller populations that experience persistent risk will be relevant in all phases of malaria control to elimination worldwide.

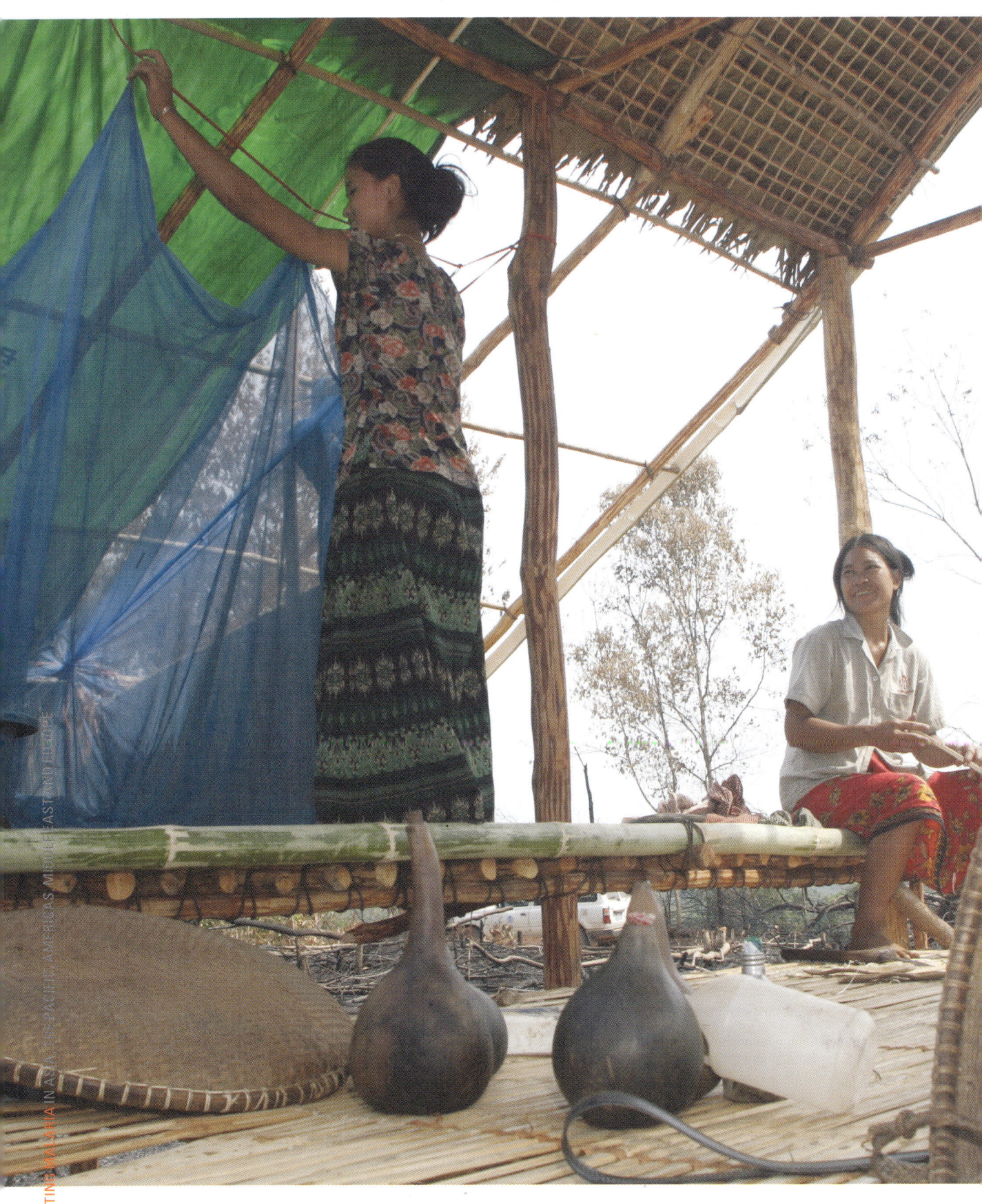

CHAPTER IX

THE WAY FORWARD

To achieve the ambitious global goals of reducing the needless loss of life due to malaria, and to further reduce the malaria burden outside of Africa, governments, development partners, and other stakeholders should focus their attention on six priority areas.

Bridge the funding gap. While more money is available for malaria control outside of Africa than ever before, these resources still fall short of the amount required for effective disease control. An unprecedented global fundraising effort is needed—mobilizing both existing and emerging donors—to ensure that all endemic countries move closer to elimination, marginalized populations are reached, and the efforts to contain drug and insecticide resistance are scaled up. It will also be critical that malaria-endemic countries benefiting from economic growth allocate more domestic resources to fight malaria, or the progress made in reducing malaria to date will be put at risk.

Increase technical assistance and knowledge transfers. To defeat malaria, many endemic countries will also need significantly more technical assistance to strengthen their malaria response. When requested, technical partners should scale up assistance to ministries of health to support them in their efforts to design, evaluate, and update national malaria control strategies and work plans. Development partners should continue to help ministries of health provide health worker training and strengthen human resources for health. Particular attention should be paid to the design of interventions that help vulnerable groups be reached.

Provide universal access to preventive interventions. Greater efforts are needed to provide protection to all those at risk of malaria, particularly in the most populous countries with the greatest numbers of cases and deaths. Attainment of this goal will be particularly challenging for those communities that are mobile or live in remote border areas. In some situations, novel vector control methods may be needed, such as insecticide-treated hammocks to protect those who work and sleep in forests overnight, or insecticidal mosquito coils to protect against outdoor biting mosquitoes. As prevalence rates fall and remain very low in many areas, new approaches need to be developed to tackle the last remaining cases.

Scale up diagnostic testing, treatment, and surveillance. With the 2012 launch of WHO's *T3: Test. Treat. Track* initiative, malaria-endemic countries and donors are urged to ensure that every suspected malaria case is tested, that every confirmed case is treated with a quality-assured antimalarial medicine, and that the disease is tracked through timely and accurate surveillance systems. Scaling up these three interconnected pillars will

| THE WAY FORWARD |

Figure 9.1
Trends in international funding for malaria control, 2000–2010

International funding for malaria control has risen by more than eight times since 2003 but still falls short of the amount required to achieve universal access to life-saving malaria prevention and control measures.

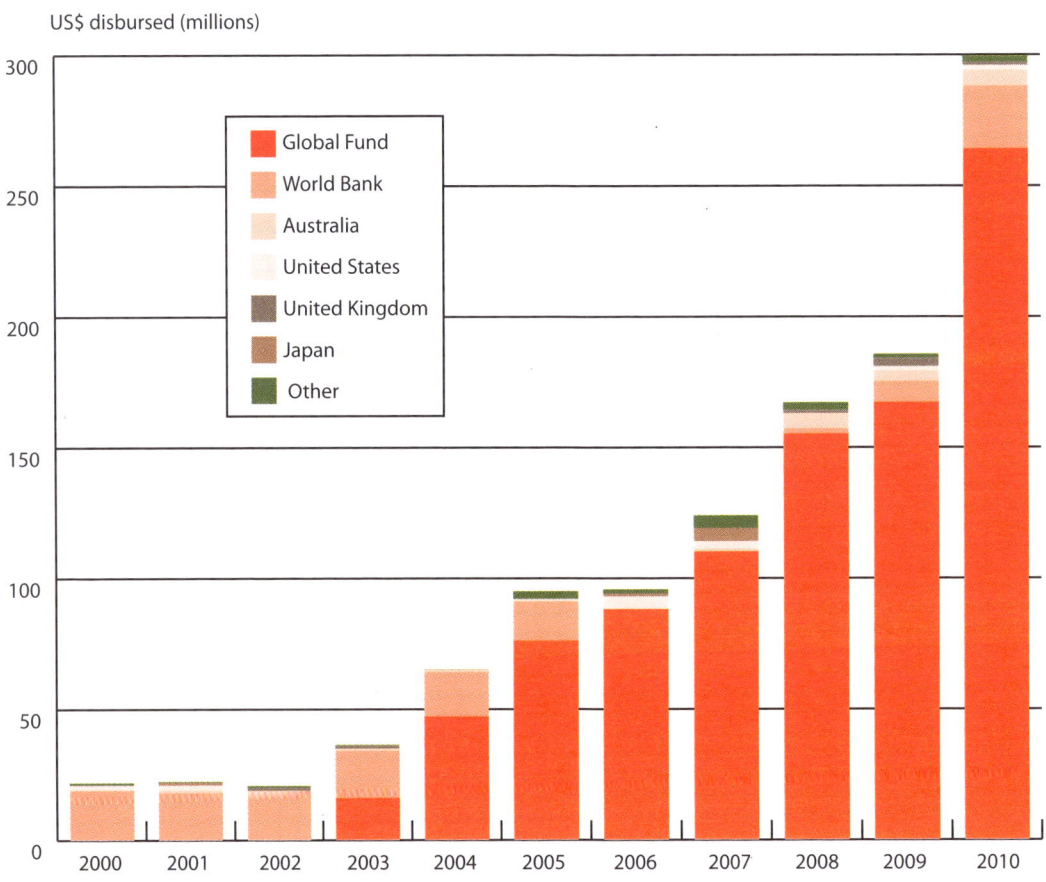

Source: World Malaria Report 2011 (*16*).

provide the much-needed bridge between efforts to achieve universal coverage with prevention tools and the goal of eliminating malaria. It will also lead to a better overall understanding of the distribution of the disease, and enable national malaria control programmes to most efficiently direct available resources to where they are needed. T3 scale-up will enable affected countries to deliver a better return on investment on malaria funding received from international donors.

Step up the fight against drug and insecticide resistance. The double threat of drug and insecticide resistance imperils recent gains in malaria prevention and control. Increased political commitment and new sources of funding will be needed to tackle these challenges. WHO has made global strategies available to address both drug and insecticide resistance. The *Global Plan for Artemisinin Resistance Containment* was released in January 2011, while the *Global Plan for Insecticide Resistance Management in Malaria Vectors* was issued in May 2012. These plans

Figure 9.2
Increase in total government spending per capita in malaria-endemic countries outside of Africa, 2000-2016

Malaria-endemic countries outside of Africa have increased total government spending between 2000–2010 and are projected to further increase spending to 2016.

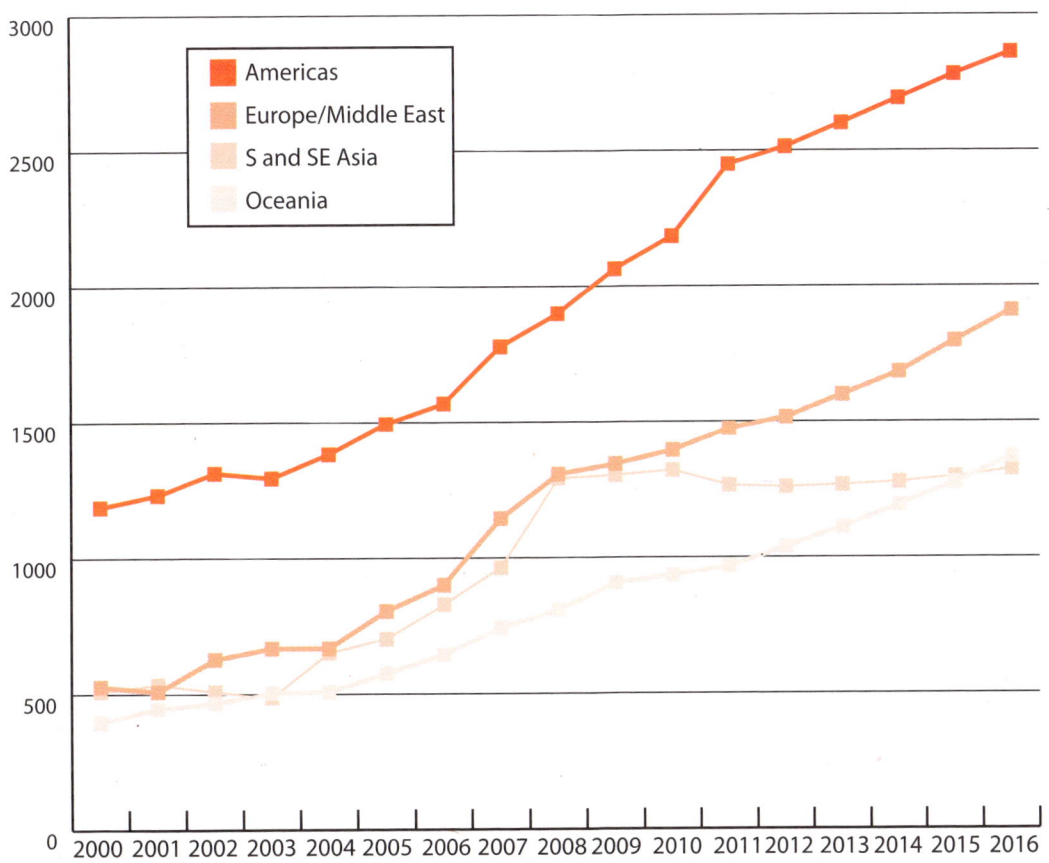

Source: World Economic Outlook, IMF, September 2011 (*39*).

should be fully implemented by governments and stakeholders in the global malaria community to preserve the current tools of malaria control until new and more effective tools become available. Contributions from the research community and industry partners will be fundamental to tackling these emerging threats.

Strengthen regional cooperation. Malaria can be defeated only if governments scale up regional cooperation efforts to strengthen the regulatory environment for pharmaceuticals and work together on removing oral artemisinin-based monotherapies and counterfeit medicines from markets. Countries also need to collaborate on managing the supply chain for malaria commodities and share information about drug and insecticide resistance patterns. In a world where malaria is increasingly confined to border areas—and where cross-border migration represents a major source

| THE WAY FORWARD |

of new malaria infection—regional cooperation is also critical for the development of cross-border strategies that are inclusive of marginalized populations.

Governments have already made a number of commitments in the UN General Assembly and the World Health Assembly, through the governing bodies of WHO regional structures,[g] and through a range of regional cooperation platforms, such as the Union of South American Nations (UNASUR) and the Association of Southeast Asian Nations (ASEAN). However, stronger political commitment will be needed to provide universal access to all key malaria interventions and to move closer to malaria elimination. With malaria designated as one of the key priorities of the UN Secretary General's five-year action agenda (2012–2017), there is an unprecedented opportunity to end the unnecessary suffering caused by this disease.

---

[g] See, for instance, the Regional Action Plan for Malaria Control and Elimination in the Western Pacific (2010–2015), which was endorsed by the 60th Regional Committee of the WHO Western Pacific Region in 2009.

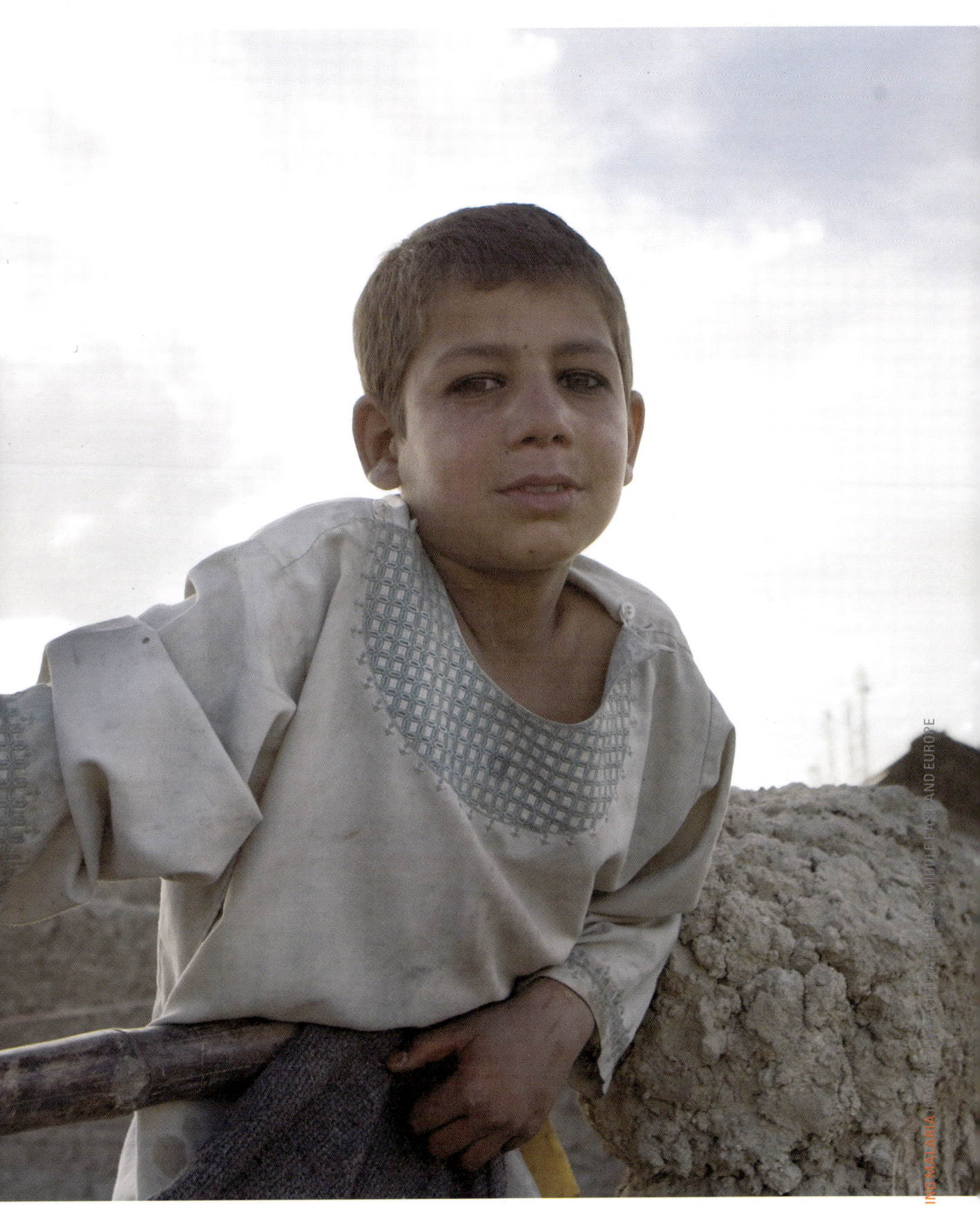

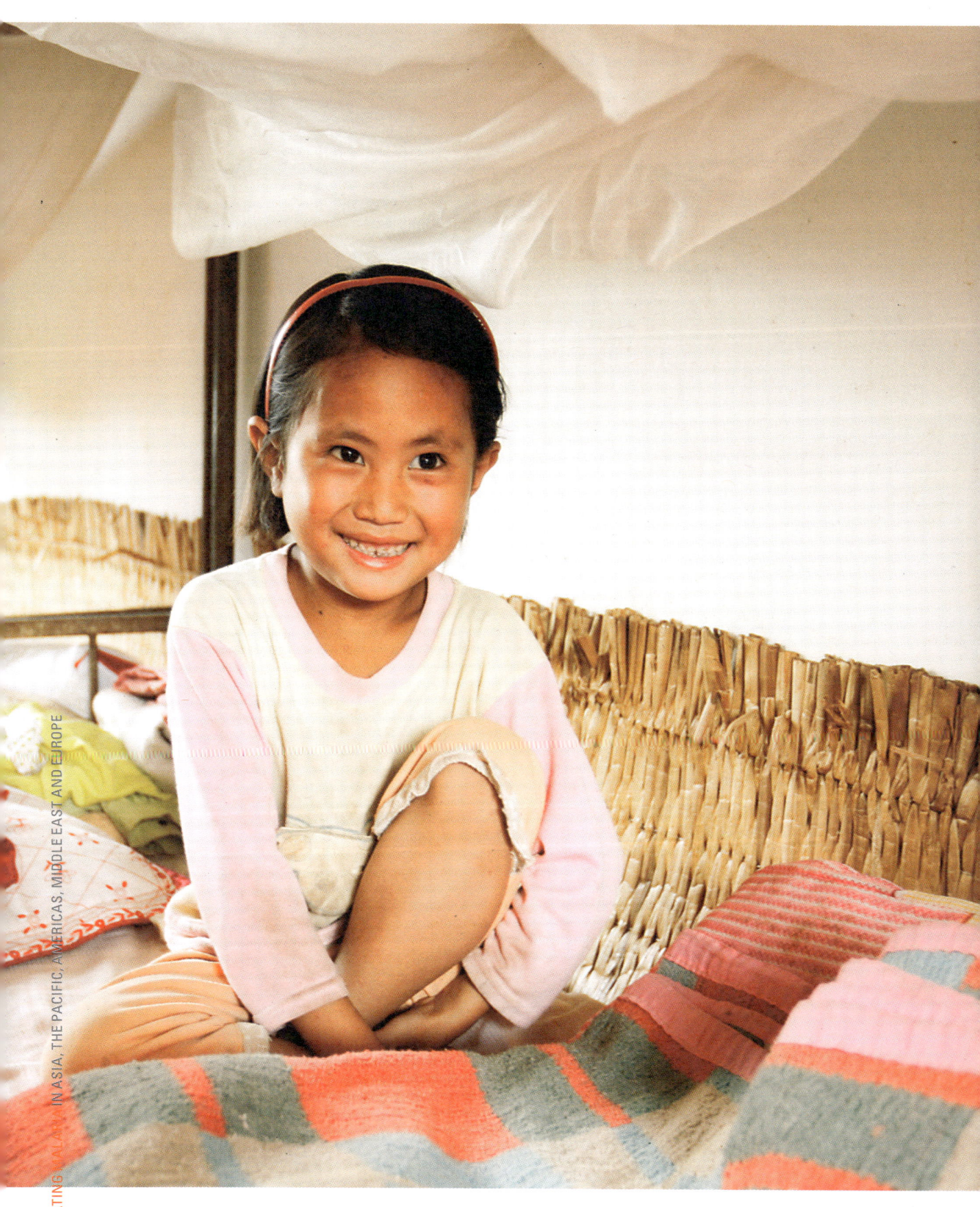

CHAPTER X

CONCLUSION

What can be gained?

The rewards for investing in malaria control and elimination—and for pursuing globally agreed-upon strategies—are potentially profound:

The burden of a senseless, avoidable tragedy can be lifted. Scaling up malaria control efforts has been proven to relieve some of the poorest, most vulnerable populations of a significant illness that causes disruption to schooling and work and, at the worst, death. Reduced illness lowers avoidable health care spending, increases productivity of workforces, provides a boost to tourism and has lasting socio-economic benefits.

Considerable financial savings can be achieved both in endemic countries and globally. Investing in the protection of the existing package of malaria control tools will result in significant savings in the long run, improving the sustainability and public health impact of malaria interventions, not only in affected countries but globally. If these efforts succeed, millions of lives can be saved and the challenges of drug and insecticide resistance can be overcome.

Health systems can be strengthened. Improving the malaria response—at both the national level and in larger regions—will boost the capacities of health systems to improve the treatment of other febrile illnesses and will help to direct financial resources where the funds are most needed. Strengthening health infrastructure and improving health information systems for malaria will strengthen countries' overall capacities to respond to future public health threats, while also helping bridge existing health inequalities.

Large areas of the world will be free from malaria in the foreseeable future. Of the 51 malaria-endemic countries outside of Africa, 17 are in the pre-elimination or elimination stage of malaria control, poised to eliminate the disease soon—removing the threat of disease from 74 million people currently at risk. Further progress requires appropriate resourcing and tight management of malaria control programmes. Yet, if elimination is attained in these countries, it would represent a historic achievement—one to be remembered for decades to come—setting the course for the eventual eradication of this ancient scourge.

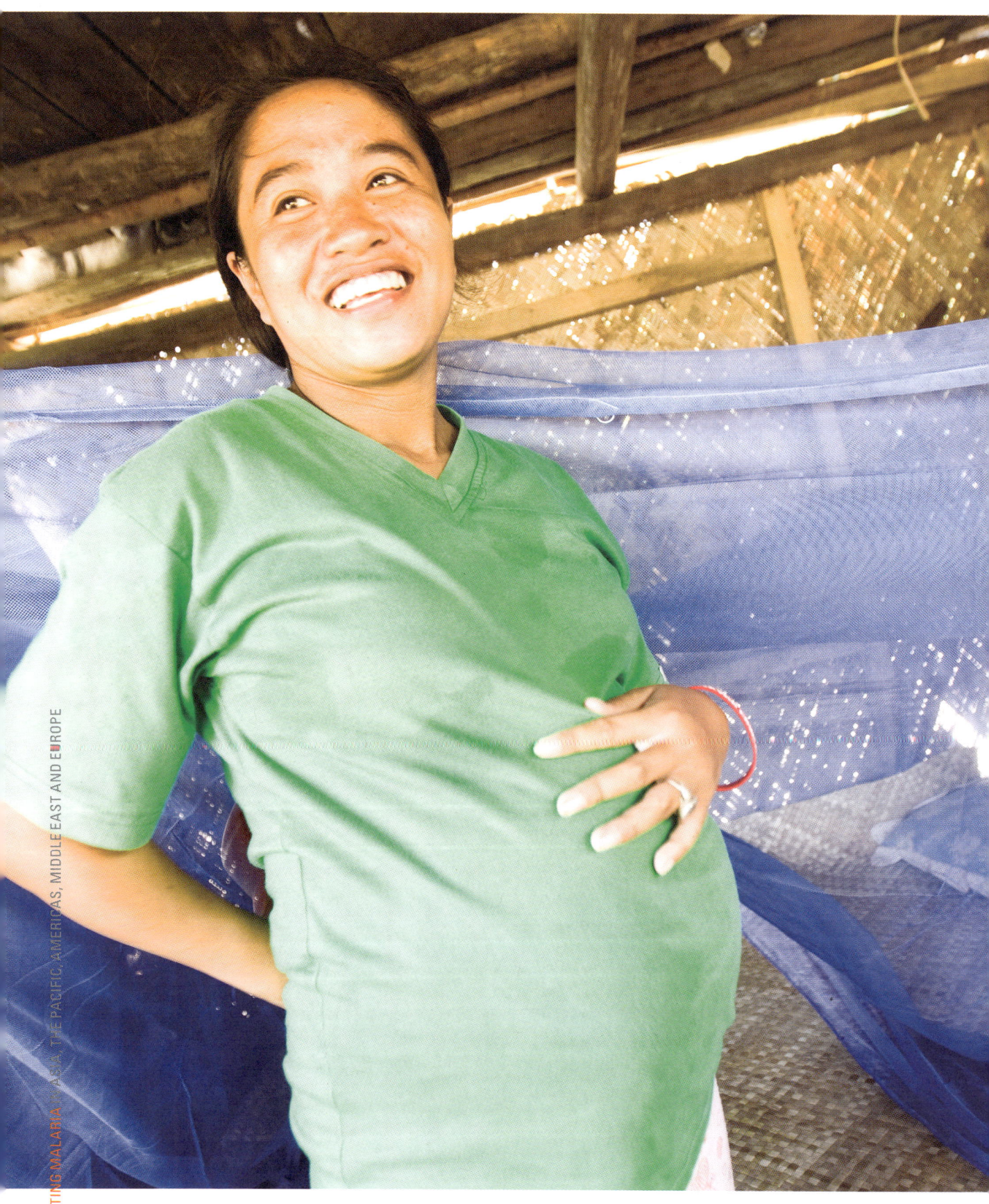

REFERENCES

1. Report of the National Commission on Macroeconomics and Health. National Commission on Macroeconomics and Health, Ministry of Health and Family Welfare, Government of India, New Delhi, August 2005.

2. Cibulskis RE, Aregawi M, Williams R, Otten M, Dye C. (2011) Worldwide Incidence of Malaria in 2009: Estimates, Time Trends, and a Critique of Methods. PLoS Med 8(12): e1001142. doi:10.1371/journal.pmed.1001142.

3. Bianca Pluess et al (2009) Malaria – a major health problem within an oil palm plantation around Popondetta, Papua New Guinea. *Malaria Journal*, 8:56.

4. *Universal access to malaria diagnostic testing: an operational manual.* Geneva, World Health Organization, 2011. http://whqlibdoc.who.int/publications/2011/9789241502092_eng.pdf.

5. Parasitological confirmation of malaria diagnosis: report of a WHO technical consultation. Geneva, World Health Organization, 2010.

6. Malaria microscopy quality assurance manual. Manila, WHO Regional Office for the Western Pacific, 2009.

7. *Results of WHO product testing of malaria RDTs: round 3 (2010–2011).* Geneva, World Health Organization, 2011. http://www.who.int/tdr/publications/documents/rdt3.pdf.

8. Foundation for Innovative New Diagnostics. *Malaria RDT product testing: interactive guide.* http://www.finddiagnostics.org/programs/malaria/find_activities/product_testing/malaria-rdt-product-testing/.

9. *Parasitological confirmation of malaria diagnosis.* Geneva, World Health Organization, 2009.

10. S Hoyer, personal communication.

11. Okell LC et al. Submicroscopic infection in Plasmodium falciparum-endemic populations: a systematic review and meta-analysis. *Journal of Infectious Diseases*, 2009, 200:1509–1517.

12. Cerruti C Jr. et al. Epidemiologic aspects of the malaria transmission cycle in an area of very low incidence in Brazil. *Malaria Journal*, 2007, 6:33.

13. Rajakaruna RS et al. Pre-elimination stage of malaria in Sri Lanka: assessing the level of hidden parasites in the population. *Malaria Journal*, 2010, 9:25.

14. Guerra CA, Gikandi PW, Tatem AJ, Noor AM, Smith DL, et al. (2008) *The Limits and Intensity of Plasmodium falciparum Transmission: Implications for Malaria Control and Elimination Worldwide.* PLoS Med 5(2): e38. doi:10.1371/journal.pmed.0050038.

15. Guerra CA, Howes RE, Patil AP, Gething PW, Van Boeckel TP, Temperley WH, Kabaria CW, Tatem AJ, Manh BH, Elyazar IRF, Baird JK, Snow RW, Hay SI (2010) *The International Limits and Population at Risk of Plasmodium vivax Transmission in 2009* PLoS Negl Trop Dis 4(8): e774. doi:10.1371/journal.pntd.0000774.

16. *World Health Organization (2011) World Malaria Report 2011*, Geneva, World Health Organization.

17. Gething, P.W., Elyazar, I.R.F., Moyes, C.L., Smith, D.L., Battle, K.E., Guerra, C.A., Patil, A.P., Tatem, A.J., Howes, R.E., Myers, M.F., George, D.B., Horby, P., Wertheim, H.F.L., Price, R.N., Müeller, I., Baird, J.K., Hay, S.I. (2012) *A long neglected world malaria map: Plasmodium vivax endemicity in 2010.* PLoS Neglected Tropical Diseases, in press.

18. Gething, P.W., Patil, A.P., Smith, D.L., Guerra, C.A., Elyazar, I.R.F., Johnston, G.L., Tatem, A.J. and Hay, S.I. (2011) A new world malaria map: Plasmodium falciparum endemicity in 2010. *Malaria Journal*, 10, 378.

REFERENCES

19. WHO (2005) *Malaria control in complex emergencies: an inter-agency field handbook.* Geneva, World Health Organization.

20. Sinka, E.M., Bangs, M.J., Manguin, S., Rubio-Palis, Y., Chareonviriyaphap, T., Coetzee, M., Mbogo, C.M., Hemingway, J., Patil, A.P., Temperley, W.H., Gething, P.W., Katarina, C.W., Burkot, T.R., Harbach, R.E., Hay, S.I. (2012) *A global map of dominant malaria vectors.* Parasites and Vectors, 5: 69.

21. Kondrashin AV (1992) Malaria in the WHO South-East Asia region. Indian J Malariol. 29:129-60.

22. Incardona S, Vong S, Chiv L, Lim P, Nhem S, Sem R, Khim N, Doung S, Mercereau-Puijalon O, Fandeur T (2007) Large-scale malaria survey in Cambodia: novel insights on species distribution and risk factors. *Malaria Journal.* 6:37.

23. Sharma SK, Tyagi PK, Padhan K, Upadhyay AK, Haque MA, Nanda N, Joshi H, Biswas S, Adak T, Das BS, Chauhan VS, Chitnis CE, Subbarao SK. *Epidemiology of malaria transmission in forest and plain ecotype villages in Sundargarh District, Orissa, India.* Trans R Soc Trop Med Hyg, 100 (2006), pp. 917–925.

24. Pluess B, Mueller I, Levi D, King G, Smith TA, Lengeler C. (2009) Malaria—a major health problem within an oil palm plantation around Popondetta, Papua New Guinea. *Malaria Journal* 8:56.

25. WHO (2010) World Malaria Report 2010. Geneva. *World Malaria Report.*

26. Bhutan Ministry of Health, Bhutan National Malaria Control Strategy 2008-2013, 2008, Vector-borne Disease Control Program: Bhutan.

27. World Health Organization. *Bhutan Malaria Control Programme Review: A Report.* WHO-SEA-MAL-264, 2010, 1-59.

28. Yangzom T, Smith Gueye C, Namgay R, Galappaththy GNL, Thimasarn K, Gosling R, Murugasampillay S, Dev V. Malaria control in Bhutan: a case study of a country embarking on elimination. *Malaria Journal*, 2012, 11(9). doi: 10.1186/1475-2875-11-9.

29. Crossette B. *Bhutan: When Environment Drives Public Health Policies*, Disease Control Priorities Project 2007. http://www.dcp2.org/features/45.

30. Ministry of Health, Royal Government of Bhutan: *Annual Health Bulletin*, 2010 Ministry of Health; 2010, 1-114.

31. National Statistical Bureau, Royal Government of Bhutan: *Bhutan at a Glance* [http://www.nbs.gov.bt/index.php?id=15].

32. VDCP, Bhutan National Strategic Plan 2012-2016. 2011, Vector-borne Disease Control Program: Bhutan.

33. Dev V. Strengthening the capacity of Bhutan malaria control programme in response to epidemics with particular emphasis on vector surveillance and cross-border activities. 2010, World Health Organization, Geneva: *Assignment Report* TRL53651.

34. Manguin S, Carnevale P, Mouchet J (2008) Biodiversity of Malaria in the World. Esther, United Kingdom, John Libbey Eurotext Limited.

35. *PAHO (2008) Report on the situation of malaria in the Americas.* Washington DC. Pan American Health Organization.

36. Sinka, M.E., Bangs, M.J, Manguin, S., Chareonviriyaphap, T., Patil, A.P., Temperley, W.H., Gething, P.W., Elyazar, I.R.F., Kabaria, C.W., Harbach, R.E. and Hay, S.I. (2011). *The dominant Anopheles vectors of human malaria in the Asia-Pacific region: occurrence data, distribution maps and bionomic précis.* Parasites and Vectors, 4: 89.

37. Cohen J (2012) Malaria resurgence: a systematic review and assessment of its causes. *Malaria Journal*, 11:122.

38. World Health Organization (2005) *Malaria control in complex emergencies an inter-agency field handbook*, Geneva, World Health Organization.

39. World Economic Outlook 2011. International Monetary Fund, Washington DC.

Briefing for policy-makers

ROLL BACK MALARIA PARTNERSHIP

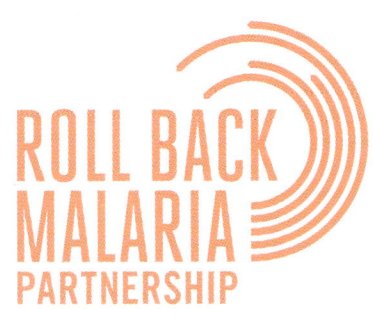

PROGRESS & IMPACT SERIES

Number 9 · November 2012

Defeating malaria in Asia, the Pacific, Americas, Middle East and Europe

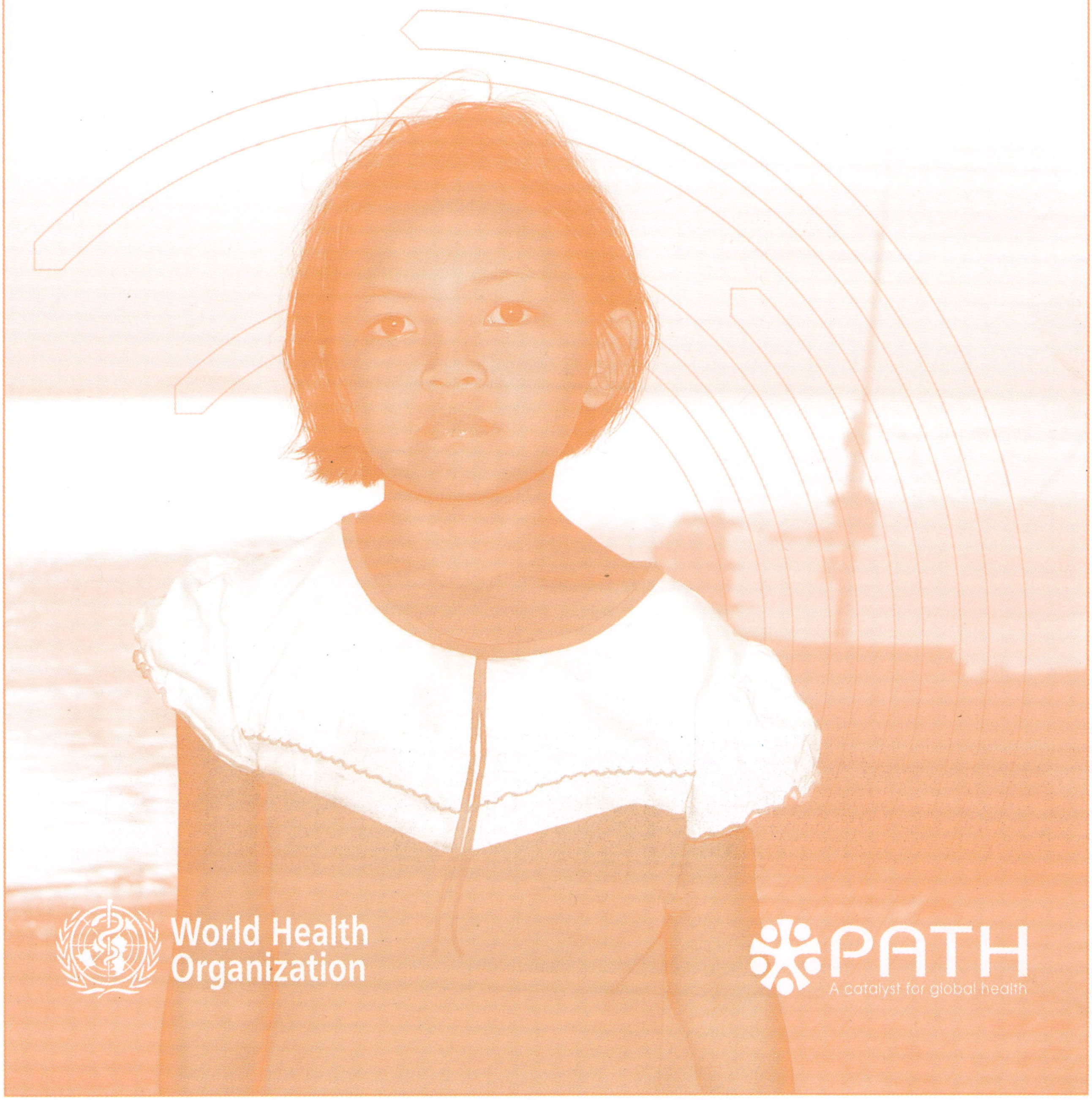

World Health Organization

PATH
A catalyst for global health

WHO Library Cataloguing-in-Publication Data

Defeating malaria in Asia, the Pacific, Americas, Middle East and Europe.
(Progress & Impact Series, n. 9)

    2 v.

    Contents: v. 1: Briefing for policy-makers -- v. 2: Technical report

1.Malaria - prevention and control. 2.Malaria - epidemiology. 3.International cooperation. 4.Asia. 5.Pacific Islands. 6.Americas. 7.Middle East. 8.Europe. I.Global Partnership to Roll Back Malaria. II.Series.

ISBN 978 92 4 150443 0   (NLM classification: WC 765)

© 2012 World Health Organization on behalf of the Roll Back Malaria Partnership Secretariat

All rights reserved. Requests for permission to reproduce or translate WHO publications – whether for sale or for noncommercial distribution – should be directed to the Roll Back Malaria (RBM) Partnership Secretariat at the address listed at the bottom of this page. Some photographs are subject to licensing fees and may not be reproduced freely; all photo enquiries should also be directed to the Secretariat.

The designations employed and the presentation of the material in this publication do not imply the expression of any opinion whatsoever on the part of the World Health Organization (WHO), the RBM Partnership Secretariat or any of its individual partners concerning the legal status of any country, territory, city or area or of its authorities, or concerning the delimitation of its frontiers or boundaries. Dotted lines on maps, where present, represent approximate border lines for which there may not yet be full agreement.

The data provided in this report were assembled from 2000 through 2011. Due to the constant updating of intervention coverage and the information supplied by countries and agencies, some numbers in this report may have since changed for this time interval; not all numbers are adjusted to a single date. However, such changes are generally minor and do not, at the time of publication, affect the overall picture of malaria intervention coverage and observed or estimated impact.

The mention or appearance in photographs of certain manufacturers and/or their products does not imply that they are endorsed or recommended by WHO, the RBM Partnership Secretariat or any of its individual partners in preference to others of a similar nature that are not mentioned.

Although every effort has been made to ensure accuracy, the information in this publication is being distributed without warranty of any kind, either expressed or implied. In no event shall WHO, the Secretariat or any of its individual partners be liable for any damages incurred arising from its use.

The named authors alone are responsible for the views expressed in this publication.

Maps | Ryan Williams, WHO Global Malaria Programme | Florence Rusciano, WHO Public Health Information and Geographic Information Systems.

Photo credits | Front cover: © Zoltan Balogh/WHO

Enquiries | Roll Back Malaria Partnership Secretariat | Hosted by the World Health Organization | Avenue Appia 20 | 1211 Geneva 27 | Switzerland | Tel.: +41 22 791 5869 | Fax: +41 22 791 1587 | E-mail: inforbm@who.int

Designed by ENLASO | Printed in France

CONTENTS

Acknowledgements 4

Foreword 5

Introduction 6

   Box 1: Tools to prevent and treat malaria outside of Africa 7

Malaria control as a development challenge 7

Malaria outside of Africa 10

Emerging threats and obstacles to progress 13

What needs to be done? 17

Conclusion 19

References 20

ACKNOWLEDGEMENTS

This report was prepared under the auspices of the Roll Back Malaria (RBM) Partnership to help assess progress towards targets set out in the Global Malaria Action Plan and the Millennium Development Goals.

This report was co-authored by Richard Cibulskis and Zsofia Szilagyi of the World Health Organization (WHO) Global Malaria Programme. Maps were produced by Ryan Williams of the WHO Global Malaria Programme and Florence Rusciano of the WHO Public Health Information and Geographic Information Systems.

The authors thank the following people for their managerial support and their work on the production of the report: Cristina Herdman (the Malaria Control and Evaluation Partnership in Africa [MACEPA], a programme at PATH) was the production manager and lead editor; Manny Lewis (MACEPA) provided editorial, proofreading, and production support; Laurent Bergeron (RBM Partnership Secretariat) assisted with report production; and Scott Brown (PATH) assisted with graphic design. The authors are also grateful to Clare Courtney, Michel Smitall, and Prudence Smith of the RBM Partnership Secretariat for their support in the release and dissemination of the report.

The RBM Progress & Impact Series Oversight Committee members are: Alexandra Farnum (chair), Suprotik Basu, Valentina Buj, John Paul Clark, Alan Court, Alexandra Fullem, Lisa Goldman, Bremen Leak, Eric Mouzin, Robert Newman, and Richard Steketee.

The report's development and production was funded in part by a grant from the Bill & Melinda Gates Foundation to PATH.

The authors are responsible for any errors and omissions.

FOREWORD

Malaria is a resilient foe. With 3.3 billion people at risk of infection globally, the disease continues to be a major burden on health systems in poor countries. Outside of Africa, malaria inflicts the heaviest toll in the Asia-Pacific.

The World Health Organization (WHO) has reported around 34 million cases of malaria in regions outside of Africa in 2010 causing 46 000 deaths. India remains by far the most affected, but rates are also high in Indonesia, Pakistan, Myanmar, Solomon Islands, and Papua New Guinea.

Beyond the human toll, malaria's economic costs include health-care expenses and diminished productivity.

The Asia-Pacific has experienced rapid economic growth over the last decade. Regional cooperation is reducing barriers between countries. There is recognition across the Asia-Pacific that working collectively is the best way to address common challenges. Malaria is one such problem.

The emergence of artemisinin resistance in Cambodia, Thailand, Myanmar, and Viet Nam is a worldwide public health risk. Failure to contain drug-resistant malaria in Asia could trigger its spread throughout the world. This would lead to a surge in cases and deaths, and undermine global progress in malaria control.

We are witnessing a growing regional emergency requiring a well-coordinated response.

The Australian Government is committed to malaria control and elimination in the Asia-Pacific. We are working with our partners—governments, civil society, international organizations, such as WHO—to address the effects of malaria on the world's most vulnerable. Together, we are working towards a strengthened regional response to artemisinin resistance.

Given the unique patterns of malaria in the Asia-Pacific, we welcome initiatives to review the challenges and opportunities for controlling and eliminating this disease. This *Briefing for policy-makers*, together with its companion piece, will contribute to our understanding of malaria-related priorities for the coming years.

Bob Carr
Minister for Foreign Affairs, Australia

| BRIEFING FOR POLICY-MAKERS |

Introduction

While the African continent carries the major burden of malaria, the disease also affects 51 countries in other parts of the world. There are 20 countries with ongoing malaria transmission in the WHO South-East Asia and Western Pacific regions, 21 countries in the Region of the Americas, and 10 in the Eastern Mediterranean and European regions. Outside of Africa, a total of 2.5 billion people are at risk of the disease, with 640 million being at high risk.

In 2010, there were an estimated 34 million malaria cases outside of Africa, and the disease caused approximately 46 000 deaths.[a] Countries in Asia and the Pacific (i.e. the WHO South-East Asia and Western Pacific regions) carry the biggest disease burden, with an estimated 88% of cases and 91% of malaria-related deaths (1). India, Indonesia, Pakistan, Myanmar, and Papua New Guinea have the highest malaria incidence.

Over the last decade, the global malaria landscape changed dramatically, and malaria received worldwide recognition as a priority public health issue. The increased availability of international funding—primarily through the Global Fund to Fight AIDS, Tuberculosis and Malaria—enabled ministries of health to vastly expand their malaria control operations. Delivery mechanisms have been established for mass distribution of conventional insecticide-treated nets (ITNs) and long-lasting insecticidal nets (LLINs); indoor residual spraying (IRS) programmes have been consolidated; and diagnostic testing, treatment, and surveillance have been scaled up (Box 1).

As a result, malaria mortality rates have decreased by 30% in countries outside of Africa, and 34 of the 51 countries have reduced their cases by more than 50%. Many countries are now on target to reach the malaria-related Millennium Development Goals and the World Health Assembly target of reducing malaria cases by at least 75% by 2015. The scale-up of interventions has not only lowered malaria-induced morbidity and mortality in many countries, but allowed ministries of health to reorient their programmes from the goal of controlling malaria to the goal of eliminating the disease altogether.

Established in 1998 by WHO, UNICEF, the United Nations Development Programme, and the World Bank, the Roll Back Malaria (RBM) Partnership serves as the overall umbrella for global malaria control efforts, aligning hundreds of partners behind a common strategy to end malaria deaths. The RBM Global Malaria Action Plan, launched in 2008, provides a global framework for action, facilitating collaboration and coordination among different partners. During the past decade, the RBM Partnership has built political commitment, improved endemic countries' access to funding, and ensured that WHO policies and recommendations for prevention, diagnosis, and treatment of malaria are widely disseminated to partners.

Despite the successes of malaria control outside of Africa, the disease continues to be a major burden not only on individuals and families, but also on national health systems, requiring constant vigilance and tailored control strategies for different geographical areas within countries. It continues to be a barrier to economic development, tourism, and foreign investment. The fight against malaria is further complicated by growing parasite resistance to antimalarial drugs and emerging mosquito resistance to insecticides. If these threats are not contained, they could undermine global malaria control efforts and reverse the impressive gains made in the last decade.

This *Briefing for policy-makers* and its companion document, a detailed analytical report, shed light on the most urgent challenges for malaria control and elimination in affected regions outside of Africa. The brief is intended for high-level decision-makers in governments, as well as for donor organizations and partners in the global malaria community.

---

[a] The uncertainty range for malaria cases outside of Africa is 32 to 45 million, while for malaria deaths it is 42 000 to 70 000.

Box 1: Tools to prevent and treat malaria outside of Africa

Countries can control malaria and move toward eliminating the disease through a multi-pronged strategy focused on achieving high coverage of vector control interventions and expanding access to diagnostic testing and quality-assured artemisinin-based combination therapies (ACTs). LLINs have been found to reduce malaria incidence by 50% in a diverse range of settings, significantly reducing unnecessary treatment costs.

- Delivering an LLIN that protects two people for three years costs US$ 1.25 per person per year.

- Large IRS programmes cost approximately US$ 2.50 or less per person protected per year.

- The cost of a rapid diagnostic test (RDT) is approximately US$ 0.60.

- The average price of a three-day course of ACT is US$ 0.50 for children, and less than US$ 1.50 for adults (1).

Malaria control as a development challenge

Following successful elimination campaigns in most of the northern hemisphere in the 1950s and 1960s, malaria is now a disease primarily affecting low and lower-middle income countries. The distribution of malaria overlaps with the global map of poverty (Figure 1) and, within endemic countries, poor and vulnerable communities are impacted more severely than others. Controlling and eliminating malaria is therefore very much a development challenge—one that is inextricably linked with poverty reduction and infrastructure development as well as health system strengthening.

Poverty is both a cause and consequence of malaria

Given the treatment costs and the financial losses resulting from work absenteeism, malaria imposes a substantial burden on individuals and affected families. The disease causes disruption to schooling and reduces the days worked not only of the sufferers but of those who care for them. For example, a single episode of malaria in India has been found to reduce the number of days worked in a household by 13, while the estimated overall monetary losses (income losses together with treatment expenses) could amount to between 200 and 400 Indian rupees (US$ 3.50 to 7.00) (2).

With an estimated 22.5 million malaria cases in India (3), this translates to an annual cost of US$ 79 to 157 million, or 0.01% of gross domestic product each year.[b] In states with the highest incidence rates, such as Chhattisgarh, Jharkhand, Meghalaya, Mizoram, and Orissa, the annual cost of illness represents more than 0.1% of a state's domestic product. The poorest 10% of the Indian population rely on sales of their assets or on borrowing to pay for health-care services, reducing a family's ability to access basic goods and affecting their long-term economic prospects.

---

[b] The uncertainty range for malaria cases in India is 17 to 30 million.

| BRIEFING FOR POLICY-MAKERS |

Figure 1
Malaria and poverty
Countries with higher proportions of their population living in poverty (less than US$ 1.25 per day) have higher death rates from malaria.

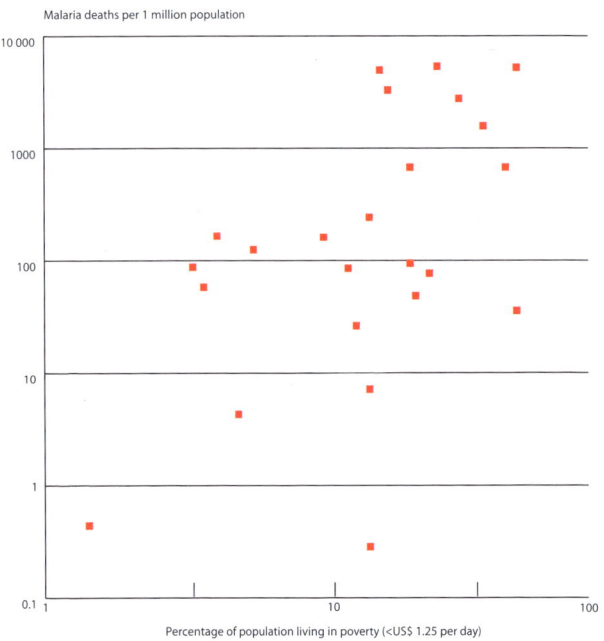

Note: This illustrative figure shows the poverty and malaria mortality rates for 24 malaria-endemic countries outside of Africa.
Source of poverty data: Human Development Report 2011.
Source of malaria mortality rates: World Malaria Report 2011.

The malaria burden also exacts a significant economic cost on societies. Businesses in endemic regions incur costs from preventing, diagnosing, and treating malaria, and register financial losses due to work absenteeism and reduced productivity. The disease discourages tourism investments and markets may remain underdeveloped owing to traders' unwillingness to travel to and invest in businesses located in malaria-endemic areas. At the same time, the combined effect of these factors further limits economic growth in some of the poorest regions.

Because their economies are less developed, many malaria-endemic countries have weak and under-resourced health systems, and public health spending tends to remain significantly below the private, out-of-pocket spending on health care. In the five countries most affected by malaria outside of Africa—India, Indonesia, Pakistan, Myanmar, and Papua New Guinea—the annual per capita government expenditure on health is less than US$ 32 per year. In Myanmar, it is US$ 2 per year, while in Pakistan, it is US$ 7 per year.[c]

Health systems in many endemic countries are characterized by the existence of long-standing health inequalities, with life expectancy and access to health services depending heavily on people's ethnicity, societal position, education, gender, age, and geographical location. Disease

[c] Figures reflect data for 2009. *World Health Statistics 2011*, Geneva, World Health Organization, 2012, p. 137.

surveillance and health information systems tend to be weak, and most malaria-endemic countries do not have well-functioning birth and death registration systems. Of the 51 endemic countries outside of Africa, 19 do not produce cause-of-death statistics at all (4).

The fight against malaria is also rendered difficult by weak pharmaceutical regulation, the wide availability of oral artemisinin-based monotherapies (and other antimalarials that do not meet international quality standards), and a lack of adequate access to quality-assured ACTs. All these factors are important drivers of drug resistance.

Given their resource constraints and weak health systems, most endemic countries lack adequate funding to deliver prevention tools or access to treatment to all populations at risk. Thus, impoverished populations are denied access to essential interventions that can prevent or cure malaria. While the number of conventional ITNs and LLINs delivered outside of Africa rose seven-fold from 2003 to 2010, only 125 million of the 640 million people at high risk of the disease were protected through vector control interventions in 2010.

Malaria affects vulnerable groups disproportionately

As malaria is beaten back in countries outside of Africa, it is becoming increasingly concentrated in marginalized population groups, including poor and rural communities; ethnic, religious, and political minorities; and communities living in hard-to-reach areas and border regions.

These communities often lack access to health care, and are difficult to reach with mass bednet distribution campaigns or public awareness campaigns about the dangers of malaria. Statistics reveal that the disease burden affects these groups disproportionately. For example, tribal communities in India constitute only 8% of the total population but they contribute 25% of the total malaria cases.

For some of these groups, access to formal health care and preventive measures may be more difficult due to language barriers or traditional beliefs. It is also often more difficult, and therefore more costly, to offer services to such populations due to infrastructural challenges, security concerns, or political considerations. Nevertheless, many countries offer successful examples of how extending these benefits is possible. In Cambodia, for instance, diagnostic testing for malaria was provided to remote tribal populations through the training of community health workers on the use of rapid diagnostic tests (RDTs).

Mobile populations such as migrant workers, refugees, and internally displaced people are also disproportionately affected by malaria. These populations have limited access to preventive interventions and health facilities, and often do not receive proper and timely treatment for their malaria infection. Myanmar has one of the largest internally displaced populations in Asia (approximately 340 000) (5), while Thailand has become a major destination for migrants from Cambodia, the Lao People's Democratic Republic, and Myanmar (6).

Population movement due to demographic, economic, and political pressures, and natural disasters or conflict may also push vulnerable communities to leave malaria-free areas and move into endemic zones. Asia is the region of the world most affected by sudden-onset natural disasters, and the likelihood of such events growing in number in the future is very high (6).

| BRIEFING FOR POLICY-MAKERS |

Malaria outside of Africa

The risk of malaria infection in populations outside of Africa is greatly variable. In some settings, such as parts of Papua New Guinea, transmission can be intense and individuals may be infected several times each year, experiencing "Africa-like malaria". In other areas, transmission intensity is so low that the annual risk of infection is less than 1 case per 1000 people. In some areas, infection rates are so low that individuals do not develop partial immunity against the disease, meaning that in certain climate and social conditions, malaria prevalence can rapidly increase and cause epidemics.

Outside of Africa, malaria is characterized by great diversity of malaria-transmitting mosquitoes and the fact that *Plasmodium (P.) falciparum* and *P. vivax* parasites are both prevalent. *P. falciparum* malaria—the most deadly form of the disease— is responsible for approximately 50% of cases, while *P. vivax* accounts for most of the rest. While *P. vivax* is less likely to trigger severe malaria and rarely kills, it does lead to considerable illness and work absenteeism, just like *P. falciparum*. Because it has a stage in the human liver that can be dormant for many months, *P. vivax* is more challenging to control and suppress, presenting a unique challenge to endemic countries.

In Asia and the Pacific, the malaria response is also complicated by the emergence of a zoonotic form of the disease. The first case of a human infection with *P. knowlesi* malaria—a disease known to affect macaque monkeys mainly—was reported in Malaysia in 1965. Since then, cases have been reported in Thailand, Cambodia, Viet Nam, and the Philippines as well. *P. knowlesi* malaria is often misdiagnosed, which can result in serious illness and can be fatal.

Progress in defeating malaria has been substantial

Despite the challenges, tremendous progress has been registered outside of Africa in the fight against malaria between 2000 and 2010. Malaria prevention and control interventions have been significantly scaled up (Figure 2), leading to an overall 30% decrease in malaria mortality rates. During this period, 34 countries reduced their cases by more than 50% (Figure 3).

Since 2007, four countries have been certified by WHO as free of malaria (Armenia, Morocco, Turkmenistan, and the United Arab Emirates). The WHO European Region is aiming for malaria elimination across the entire region by 2015. *P. falciparum* transmission has already been eliminated, with the last cases reported in Tajikistan in 2008. Only *P. vivax* remains, with local transmission occurring just in Azerbaijan (50 cases in 2010), Tajikistan (111 cases), and Turkey (9 cases). Georgia reported no locally acquired cases in 2010.

Argentina, El Salvador, Mexico, and Paraguay are also close to eliminating malaria and have reported few cases—mostly *P. vivax*—in recent years. Iraq reported no cases due to local transmission in 2009 and 2010. Bhutan reported only 401 cases in 2010, while Sri Lanka has reduced its number of cases from more than 200 000 in 2000 to less than 700 in 2010. Several other countries are revising their malaria control strategies to scale up efforts for nationwide elimination.

Altogether, 17 countries outside of Africa are in the pre-elimination or elimination stage of malaria control. These countries are poised to eliminate malaria in the foreseeable future, removing the threat of disease from 74 million people currently at risk. In these countries, malaria surveillance is of paramount importance and each malaria case should be investigated.

Higher-burden countries are making slower progress

Progress in reducing malaria has been slower in higher-burden countries, although some countries such as Papua New Guinea appear to be showing significant progress in reducing

Figure 2
Prevention, testing, and treatment coverage outside of Africa, 2000–2010

There have been large increases in the number of bednets (conventional ITNs and LLINs) delivered, while RDTs and ACT treatment courses were also scaled up. The number of people protected by IRS has not changed significantly.

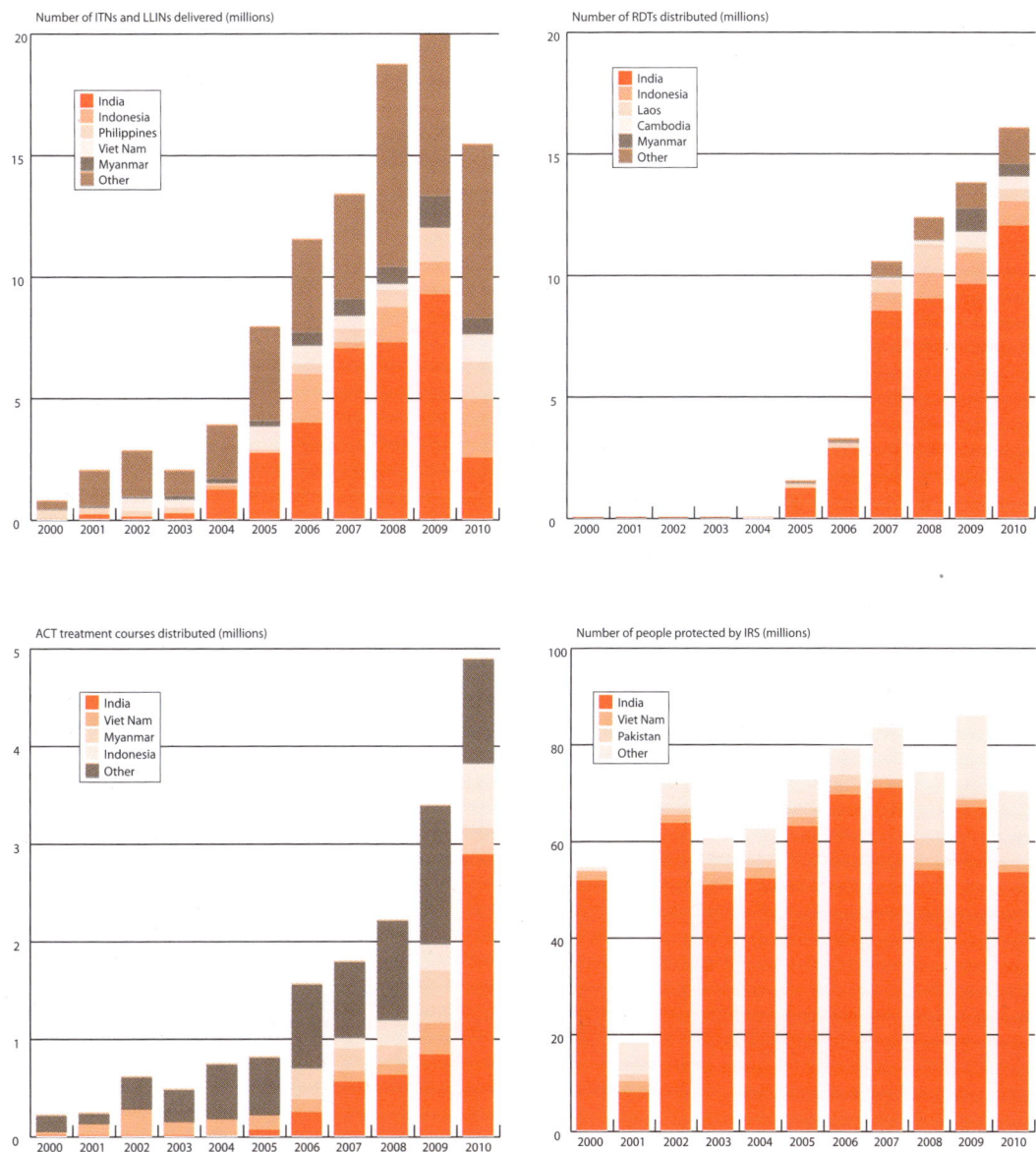

Source: World Malaria Report 2011, World Health Organization, 2011.

| BRIEFING FOR POLICY-MAKERS |

Figure 3
Reductions in malaria cases worldwide
A total of 34 countries outside of Africa have reduced cases by more than 50% since 2000; another 4 have reduced cases by 25% or more.

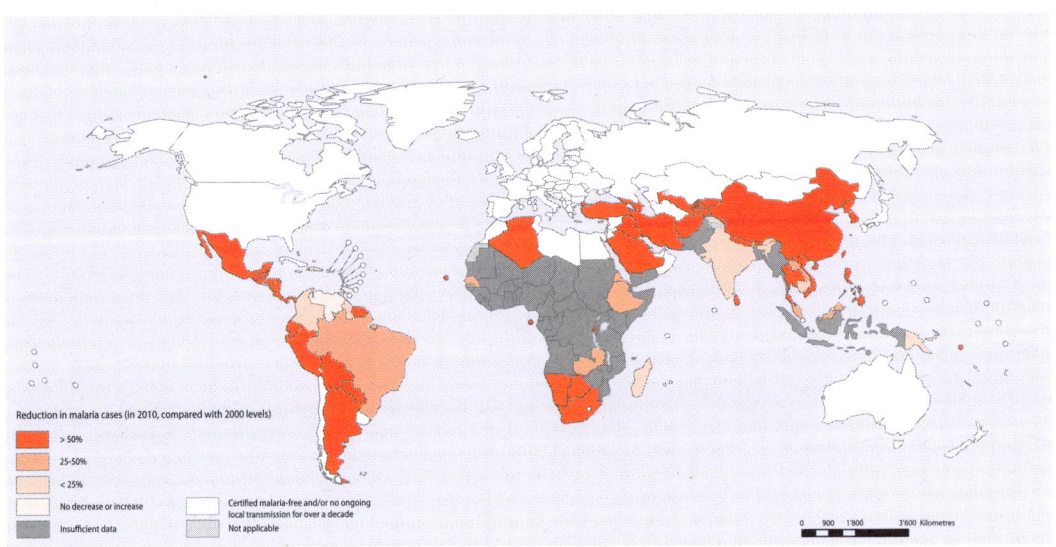

Source: World Health Organization, 2010.
Map production: WHO Global Malaria Programme.

parasite prevalence. Nonetheless, India, Indonesia, Myanmar, Pakistan, and Papua New Guinea still account for a relatively high number of cases and deaths. The slower progress may be related to smaller per capita investments in malaria control, as well as the difficulties of operating control programmes on a large scale.

Higher-burden countries will therefore need substantial financial resources and technical assistance to strengthen their health systems before they can visibly improve their malaria response. At their current pace, it is unlikely that they can achieve the malaria-specific Millennium Development Goals and the World Health Assembly target of reducing the malaria burden by at least 75% by 2015. Further progress cannot be attained without high-level political commitment and tight management of malaria control programmes.

P. vivax is more challenging to control

As malaria control programmes are intensified, the number of *P. falciparum* cases declines faster than that of *P. vivax*, requiring substantial adjustments to malaria control strategies.

P. vivax malaria is more challenging to control because the parasite is tolerant of a wider range of environmental conditions and can be transmitted by mosquitoes even before infected people develop symptoms. It is also more difficult to treat because the parasite may develop a dormant form residing in the liver. An individual infected with *P. vivax* may remain asymptomatic for months to years and then relapse. Dormant *P. vivax* parasites cannot be detected with existing diagnostic tests, meaning there may be a large reservoir of infected people who are unaware of their condition and are not counted in malaria surveillance systems until they relapse.

Another difficulty in treating *P. vivax* malaria is that liver-stage parasites can only be eliminated through a 14-day course of primaquine, which can produce serious side effects (hemolytic anaemia) in patients who have more severe forms of glucose-6-phosphate dehydrogenase (G6PD) deficiency. Testing for G6PD deficiency is currently technically challenging and relatively expensive; hence, many clinicians do not prescribe primaquine when the risk from taking the drug may exceed that from the disease.

As disease incidence decreases, populations are more prone to epidemics

As the incidence of malaria is reduced, naturally acquired partial immunity to the disease decreases. Although new infections are less likely to occur, they can rapidly lead to illness, which can be severe, and can more easily spread via the mosquito vector from one person to another. If control programmes are weakened or abandoned, devastating outbreaks or epidemics can strike unsuspecting populations. The vast majority of resurgences in the past 80 years (91%) have been due, at least in part, to the weakening of malaria control programmes, with resource constraints being the most commonly identified factor (57%) (7).

Epidemics also occur around traditionally endemic zones in areas where transmission has been eliminated. These outbreaks are generally associated with deteriorating social and economic conditions. In order to protect the impressive gains of the past decade, control programmes must be sustained in all malaria-prone areas, even as countries approach elimination and are certified by WHO as free of malaria.

Emerging threats and obstacles to progress

There are three major challenges that threaten the future of malaria control globally:

- The lack of adequate funding to further scale up malaria control and elimination efforts.

- Growing parasite resistance to antimalarial drugs.

- Emerging mosquito resistance to insecticides used on LLINs and in IRS programmes.

Containing drug and insecticide resistance is an urgent issue that is critical to preserving the most effective first-line therapies for uncomplicated malaria and maintaining the effectiveness of vector control interventions. WHO has issued global plans to tackle both challenges, assigning clear roles to all stakeholders, including governments, donor organizations, the research community, and industry. These strategies should be implemented in full to ensure that the massive prevention and control investments of the last decade are protected.

1. Lack of adequate financing

Since 2003, international funding for malaria control outside of Africa has risen from less than US$ 17 million in 2000 to US$ 300 million in 2010, primarily due to funding made available through the Global Fund to Fight AIDS, Tuberculosis and Malaria (Figure 4). In 2010, the Global Fund accounted for approximately 88% of international funding for malaria control outside of Africa.[d] A further 8% of international funding was derived from the World Bank and another 2% from Australia.

This increase in funding was matched in some instances by increases in domestic spending by countries such as Bangladesh and Colombia (Figure 5). In November 2011, Brazil

---

[d] The Global Fund obtains 90% of its donations from the United States, France, Germany, United Kingdom, Japan, European Commission, Canada, Italy, Bill & Melinda Gates Foundation, Spain, Netherlands, and Sweden.

| BRIEFING FOR POLICY-MAKERS |

Figure 4
Trends in international funding for malaria control outside of Africa, 2000–2010

International funding for malaria control has seen a more than eight-fold increase since 2003 but still falls short of the amount required to achieve universal access to life-saving malaria prevention and control measures.

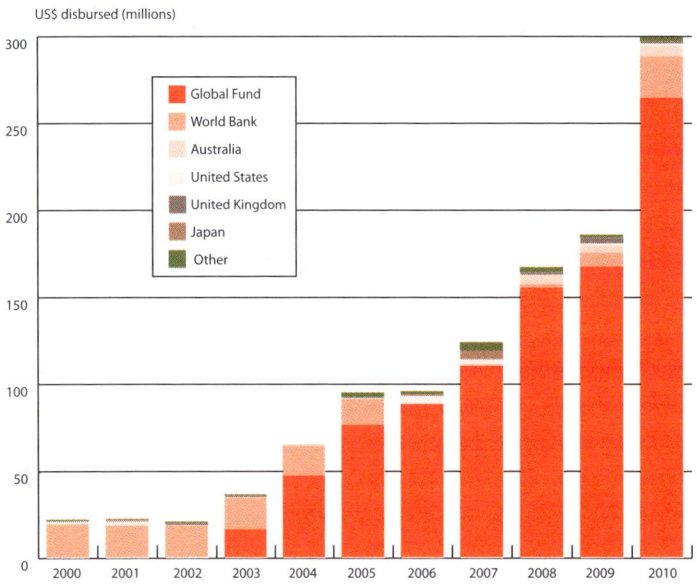

Source: World Malaria Report 2011, World Health Organization, 2011.

declined to accept funds for Phase 2 of its Round 8 Global Fund malaria grant, even though it had successfully completed Phase 1.

However, the currently available funding is inadequate to reach global malaria targets and to provide universal access to life-saving malaria prevention and control measures—a requirement estimated to be about US$ 3 billion.

If current trends persist, the overall level of international financing will decline in the coming years. The Global Fund has recently experienced lower levels of replenishment than expected and, along with other donors, is increasingly focusing its funding to the poorest countries in sub-Saharan Africa with the highest malaria burden.

Funding from domestic sources is not guaranteed either and may be threatened because of the very success of malaria control; as malaria incidence decreases, governments often shift resources to other disease areas or other development priorities. Without the necessary resources, the loftier ambitions of malaria elimination and ultimate eradication cannot be reached.

2. Containing drug resistance

Artemisinin-based combination therapies (ACTs) are critical to the future of malaria control programmes worldwide. Quality-assured ACTs are recommended by WHO as the first-line treatment for uncomplicated *P. falciparum* malaria. Expanding access to these highly effective combination therapies has contributed significantly to recent advances against malaria, but progress is now

Figure 5
Contributions to national malaria control by governments of Bangladesh and Colombia, 2000–2010
In some countries, domestic contributions for malaria control have also risen.

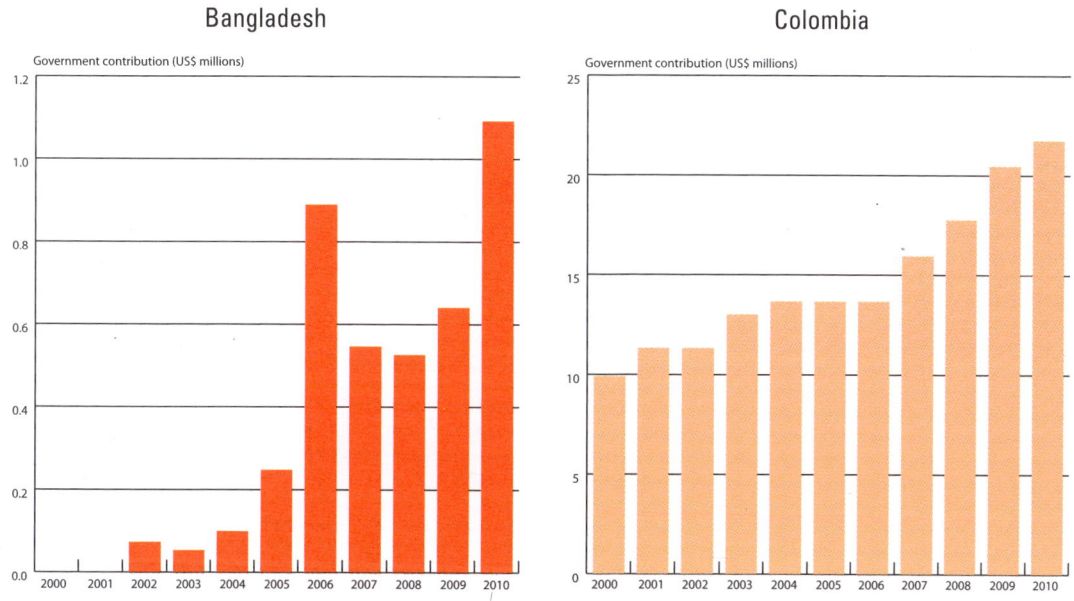

Source: World Malaria Report 2011, World Health Organization, 2011.

threatened by the emergence of artemisinin-resistant parasites in South-East Asia.

In recent years, *P. falciparum* resistance to artemisinins has been detected in four countries of the Greater Mekong subregion: Cambodia, Myanmar, Thailand, and Viet Nam. If resistance spreads to India or sub-Saharan Africa, the public health consequences could be dire, as no alternative antimalarial medicine is available with the same level of efficacy and tolerability as ACTs. Given the ever-increasing levels of population movement in Asia and the Pacific, the geographic scope of the problem could widen quickly, posing a health security risk for many countries in the region that have ongoing malaria transmission.

There is therefore a limited window of opportunity to avert a regional public health disaster, which could have severe global consequences. In January 2011, WHO released the *Global Plan for Artemisinin Resistance Containment* (GPARC), calling on all stakeholders to maximize efforts to protect the efficacy of ACTs. Despite WHO's call to action, not enough is being done. Containment efforts in the Greater Mekong subregion have been effective where implemented, but efforts need to be strengthened and expanded.

This requires considerable investment in monitoring drug efficacy, improving access to diagnostics and quality-assured ACTs, scaling up basic prevention and control interventions to reduce malaria transmission, and increasing support for, and monitoring of, mobile and migrant populations. Governments should also take targeted regulatory measures to remove oral artemisinin-based monotherapies from markets, along with antimalarials that do not meet international quality standards.

| BRIEFING FOR POLICY-MAKERS |

The Greater Mekong subregion has long been the cradle of antimalarial drug resistance, and the spread of resistant parasites to India and Africa led to a dramatic rise in the global malaria burden in previous decades. The spread—or independent emergence—of artemisinin resistance in other parts of the world could again trigger a global resurgence of malaria-related illness and death, with major social and economic costs to societies.

Drug-resistance containment has major cost implications for the public health budgets of countries in the Greater Mekong subregion, and affected countries cannot fight this challenge alone. Increased international assistance would deliver significant savings in the long run, improving the sustainability and public health impact of malaria interventions globally. Most endemic countries outside of the Greater Mekong subregion also need additional resources to implement the GPARC's recommendations and to prevent the emergence of drug resistance.

3. Managing insecticide resistance

In parallel with efforts to contain drug resistance, a coordinated response is needed to tackle emerging mosquito resistance to the insecticides used on LLINs and in IRS programmes. Existing vector control tools are still effective in the vast majority of settings, but resistance to at least one insecticide has now been reported from 64 countries with ongoing malaria transmission around the world; 24 of these countries are outside of Africa.

Insecticide resistance involves all major vector species and all classes of insecticides and has the potential to substantially weaken control programmes. Resistance to a class of chemicals known as pyrethroids seems to be the most widespread. The pyrethroids are not only highly effective, but are the least expensive of the four classes of insecticides available for public health vector control. They are the most commonly used chemicals for IRS and are currently the only class available for use on LLINs.

In May 2012, WHO released the *Global Plan for Insecticide Resistance Management in malaria vectors* (GPIRM), outlining the pillars of action required to confront and overcome this threat. The GPIRM calls on endemic countries, donor organizations, UN agencies, as well as research and industry partners, to implement a five-pillar strategy to tackle insecticide resistance and to facilitate the development of innovative vector control tools and strategies.

The five pillars are the following:

- Plan and implement insecticide resistance management strategies in malaria-endemic countries.

- Ensure proper, timely entomological and resistance monitoring and effective data management.

- Develop new, innovative vector control tools.

- Fill gaps in knowledge on mechanisms of insecticide resistance and the impact of current insecticide resistance management approaches.

- Ensure that enabling mechanisms (advocacy, human, and financial resources) are in place.

Most affected countries have not yet carried out adequate testing for insecticide resistance, which means that global understanding of the scale of insecticide resistance remains incomplete. To tackle this problem, the GPIRM also calls for the establishment of a global database on insecticide resistance to help malaria-endemic countries and donors take targeted action.

What needs to be done?

To achieve the ambitious global goals of reducing the needless loss of life due to malaria, and to further reduce the malaria burden outside of Africa, governments, development partners, and other stakeholders should focus their attention on six priority areas.

1. Bridge the funding gap. While more money is available for malaria control outside of Africa than ever before, these resources still fall short of the amount required for effective disease control. An unprecedented global fundraising effort is needed—mobilizing both existing and emerging donors—to ensure that all endemic countries move closer to elimination, marginalized populations are reached, and the efforts to contain drug and insecticide resistance are scaled up. It will also be critical that malaria-endemic countries benefiting from economic growth allocate more domestic resources to fight malaria, or the progress made in reducing malaria to date will be put at risk.

2. Increase technical assistance and knowledge transfers. To defeat malaria, many endemic countries will also need significantly more technical assistance to strengthen their malaria response. When requested, technical partners should scale up assistance to ministries of health to support them in their efforts to design, evaluate, and update national malaria control strategies and work plans. Development partners should continue to help ministries of health provide health worker training and strengthen human resources for health. Particular attention should be paid to the design of interventions that help reach vulnerable groups.

3. Provide universal access to preventive interventions. Greater efforts are needed to provide protection to all those at risk of malaria, particularly in the most populous countries with the greatest numbers of cases and deaths. Attainment of this goal will be particularly challenging for those communities that are mobile or live in remote border areas. In some situations, novel vector control methods may be needed, such as insecticide-treated hammocks to protect those who work and sleep in forests overnight, or insecticidal mosquito coils to protect against outdoor biting mosquitoes. As prevalence rates fall and remain very low in many areas, new approaches need to be developed to tackle the last remaining cases.

4. Scale up diagnostic testing, treatment, and surveillance. With the 2012 launch of WHO's *T3: Test. Treat. Track* initiative, malaria-endemic countries and donors are urged to ensure that every suspected malaria case is tested, that every confirmed case is treated with a quality-assured antimalarial medicine, and that the disease is tracked through timely and accurate surveillance systems. Scaling up these three interconnected pillars will provide the much-needed bridge between efforts to achieve universal coverage with prevention tools and the goal of eliminating malaria. It will also lead to a better overall understanding of the distribution of the disease, and enable national malaria control programmes to most efficiently direct available resources to where they are needed. T3 scale-up will enable affected countries to deliver a better return on investment on malaria funding received from international donors.

5. Step up the fight against drug and insecticide resistance. The double threat of drug and insecticide resistance imperils recent gains in malaria prevention and control. Increased political commitment and new sources of funding will be needed to tackle these challenges. WHO has made global strategies available to address both drug and insecticide resistance. The *Global Plan for Artemisinin Resistance Containment* was released in January 2011, while the *Global Plan for Insecticide Resistance Management in malaria vectors* was issued in May 2012. These plans should be fully implemented by governments and stakeholders in the global malaria community to preserve the current tools of malaria control until new and more effective tools become available.

| BRIEFING FOR POLICY-MAKERS |

Figure 6
Phases of malaria control among all malaria-endemic countries, 2011
Seventeen countries are in the pre-elimination or elimination stage of malaria control and poised to eliminate malaria, removing the threat of disease from 74 million people currently at risk.

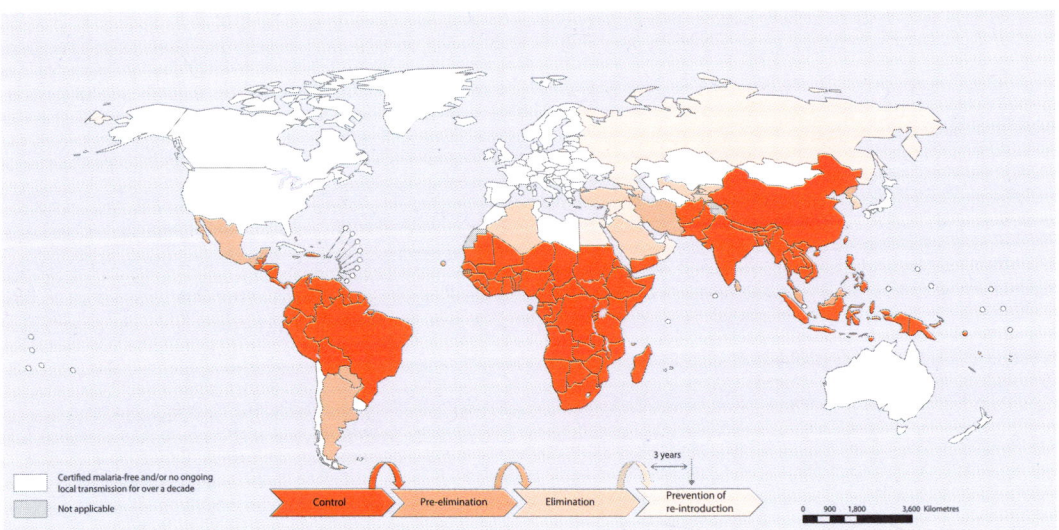

Source: World Health Organization, 2011.
Map production: WHO Global Malaria Programme.

Contributions from the research community and industry partners will be fundamental to tackling these emerging threats.

6. Strengthen regional cooperation. Malaria can be defeated only if governments scale up regional cooperation efforts to strengthen the regulatory environment for pharmaceuticals and work together on removing oral artemisinin-based monotherapies and counterfeit medicines from markets. Countries also need to collaborate on managing the supply chain for malaria commodities and share information about drug and insecticide resistance patterns. In a world where malaria is increasingly confined to border areas—and where cross-border migration represents a major source of new malaria infection—regional cooperation is also critical for the development of cross-border strategies that are inclusive of marginalized populations.

Governments have already made a number of commitments in the UN General Assembly and the World Health Assembly, through the governing bodies of WHO regional structures,[e] and through a range of regional cooperation platforms, such as the Union of South American Nations (UNASUR) and the Association of Southeast Asian Nations (ASEAN). However, stronger political commitment will be needed to provide universal access to all key malaria interventions and to move closer to malaria elimination. With malaria designated as one of the key priorities of the UN Secretary General's five-year action agenda (2012–2017), there is an unprecedented opportunity to end the unnecessary suffering caused by this disease.

What can be gained?

The rewards for investing in malaria control and elimination—and for pursuing globally agreed-upon strategies—are potentially profound:

The burden of a senseless, avoidable tragedy can be lifted. Scaling up malaria control efforts has been proven to relieve some of the poorest, most

[e] See, for instance, the Regional Action Plan for Malaria Control and Elimination in the Western Pacific (2010–2015), which was endorsed by the 60th Regional Committee of the WHO Western Pacific Region in 2009.

vulnerable populations of a significant illness that causes disruption to schooling and work and, at the worst, death. Reduced illness lowers avoidable health-care spending, increases productivity of workforces, provides a boost to tourism and has lasting socio-economic benefits.

Considerable financial savings can be achieved both in endemic countries and globally. Investing in the protection of the existing package of malaria control tools will result in significant savings in the long run, improving the sustainability and public health impact of malaria interventions, not only in affected countries but globally. If these efforts succeed, millions of lives can be saved and the challenges of drug and insecticide resistance can be overcome.

Health systems can be strengthened. Improving the malaria response—at both the national level and in larger regions—will boost the capacities of health systems to improve the treatment of other febrile illnesses and will help to direct financial resources where the funds are most needed. Strengthening health infrastructure and improving health information systems for malaria will strengthen countries' overall capacities to respond to future public health threats, while also helping bridge existing health inequalities.

Large areas of the world will be free from malaria in the foreseeable future. Of the 51 malaria-endemic countries outside of Africa, 17 are in the pre-elimination or elimination stage of malaria control, poised to eliminate the disease soon—removing the threat of disease from 74 million people currently at risk (Figure 6). Further progress requires appropriate resourcing and tight management of malaria control programmes. Yet, if elimination is attained in these countries, it would represent a historic achievement—one to be remembered for decades to come—setting the course for the eventual eradication of this ancient scourge.

Conclusion

There is an urgent need to reduce malaria incidence in higher-burden countries outside of Africa, and to help countries that are close to elimination to become certified by WHO as free of malaria. Appropriate and sustained financing is required to design and implement effective malaria control and elimination programmes that take into account the changing epidemiology of malaria and the spread of drug and insecticide resistance. To make this happen, broad political commitment is needed to implement strategies and foster partnerships that will help to achieve further progress. The malaria response will be judged in the near term by the reductions in malaria-related morbidity and mortality that are achieved, and in the long term by its durable contribution to overall health and development globally.

REFERENCES

1. *World Malaria Report 2011*. Geneva, World Health Organization, 2011.

2. *Report of the National Commission on Macroeconomics and Health*. National Commission on Macroeconomics and Health, Ministry of Health and Family Welfare, Government of India, New Delhi, August 2005.

3. Cibulskis RE, Aregawi M, Williams R, Otten M, Dye C. (2011) Worldwide Incidence of Malaria in 2009: Estimates, Time Trends, and a Critique of Methods. *PLoS Med* 8(12): e1001142. doi:10.1371/journal.pmed.1001142.

4. *World Health Statistics 2011*. Geneva, World Health Organization, 2012, p. 44.

5. *Statistical snapshot for South-East Asia, as of January 2012*. New York, UNHCR, 2012 (http://www.unhcr.org/pages/4b17be9b6.html, accessed 29 August 2012).

6. *World Migration Report 2011*. Geneva, International Organization for Migration, 2011.

7. Cohen JM, Smith DL, Cotter C, Ward A, Yamey G, Sabot OJ, Moonen B. Malaria resurgence: a systematic review and assessment of its causes. *Malaria Journal*, 2012, 11:122.